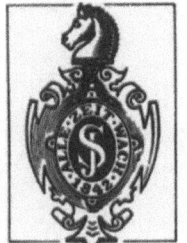

Springer-Verlag France S.A.R.L

J.-P. Homasson and N.J. Bell (Eds.)

Cryotherapy in Chest Medicine

Preface by Professor Andrew A. Gage

with 140 Figures

Springer-Verlag France S.A.R.L

Jean-Paul Homasson, M.D.
Centre Hospitalier Spécialisé en Pneumologie
24, rue A. Thuret
94669 Chevilly-Larue Cedex
France

Nicholas Bell, M.D.
3 Old Wooton Village, Boars Hill
0X15JL Oxford
United Kingdom

© Springer-Verlag France 1992
Originally published by Springer-Verlag France, Paris, 1992
Softcover reprint of the hardcover 1st edition 1992

The use of registered names, trademarks, etc. in this publication does not imply, even in the absence of a specific statement, that such names are exempt from the relevant protective laws and regulations and therefore free for general use.
Product Liability : The publisher can give no guarantee for information about drug dosage and application there of contained in this book. In every individual case the respective user must check its accuracy by consulting other pharmaceutical litterature.

ISBN 978-2-8178-0882-6   ISBN 978-2-8178-0880-2 (eBook)
DOI 10.1007/978-2-8178-0880-2

2918/3917/543210. Printed on acid free paper.

Table of contents

Preface

Cryosurgery is a method of therapy that uses freezing temperatures to achieve specific effects on tissues. Depending upon the technique of treatment, the tissue response varies from an inflammatory reaction, which is associated with a minor freezing injury, to the destructive effect which is characteristic of severe freezing injury. Cryosurgical treatments require the use of special apparatus cooled by cryogenic agents to produce the freezing temperatures necessary in the tissues. As with any other method of therapy, the physician must place emphasis on the selection of appropriate patients, on the careful determination of the nature and extent of disease, and on precise cryosurgical technique in order to achieve good results. The use of cryosurgery for the treatment of cancer requires special care to produce lethal temperatures in the lesion, especially when the goal is to cure the cancer.

The recent evolution of cryosurgery as a therapeutic technique and the rapid growth of its use in the several specialities of medicine can be attributed to the development of cryosurgical apparatus utilizing liquid nitrogen in the early 1960's. The apparatus was originally designed to produce a cryogenic lesion in the brain for the treatment of Parkinsonism and other neuromuscular disorders. However, it was obvious that the cryosurgical techniques had wider usefulness and this quickly led to trial usage in diverse diseases, including cancer, in the years 1964-1970. Most of the clinical investigations were for lesions in easily accessible sites, such as the skin and oral cavity which were areas where the treatment could be given under direct vision and the results of treatment could be viewed easily and at frequent intervals. Though endoscopic cryosurgical techniques were used for the treatment of prostatic disease and of laryngeal disease, the restricted visualization of the lesion, as well as some limitations in apparatus, precluded continued development at that time.

In the following years, some early uses of cryosurgery have fallen into disfavor, mostly because of effective competing methods of therapy, but other uses of cryosurgery have become part of standard medical practice, as demonstrated by incorporation into textbooks of surgery and its specialities. Today, the commonly accepted uses of cryosurgery are for the treatment of many types of skin disease, including cancer, for the treatment of benign and dysplastic mucosal lesions, including intraepithelial neoplasia, and for cardiac surgery in the treatment of tachyarrhythmias. Cryosurgery is mentioned in textbooks as alternative treatment for such conditions as oral cancer, anorectal cancer, bone tumor, prostatic cancer and a variety of other conditions of an inflammatory or degenerative nature affecting diverse organs and tissues. In general, visceral cryosurgery has remained largely undeveloped because of the need to obtain adequate exposure and accurate delineation of the disease.

The viability of cryosurgery as a therapeutic technique is demonstrated by the many reports which appear in the medical journals of the past recent years. The range of publications in the different specialities of medicine demonstrates that cryosurgery is progressing as new uses are described and new technology becomes available.

Improvements in cryosurgical apparatus, including the development of thin cryosurgical probes, have increased the potential scope and therapeutic applications of cryosurgery. Modern imaging techniques, including CT, MRI and ultrasound, are revising the prospects for the use of cryosurgery in visceral disease. They have substantially enhanced the ability to delineate the extent of the disease and plan the cryosurgical treatment. The use of ultrasound as an intraoperative monitoring device during cryosurgery has facilitated the present-day applications of cryosurgery to hepatic and prostatic cancer.

The use of cryosurgery for tracheobronchial and lung disease represents a new frontier in which the emphasis is on the techniques of endoscopic tracheobronchial cryosurgery. Since competitive techniques, such as laser therapy, are effective in this therapeutic field, careful description of the place of cryosurgery in terms of indications for use, techniques and results is required. This textbook meets that need. We are indebted to the editors of the book and to the authors of its chapters for producing a text which provides the fundamental basis for further work to develop the use of cryosurgery in chest medicine.

Andrew A. Gage, M.D.
Professor of Surgery
School of Medicine and Biomedical Sciences
SUNY at Buffalo
Deputy Institute Director
Roswell Park Cancer Institute

Acknowledgements

The contributors would like to thank Eutherapie Laboratory who helped with the production of the colour illustrations in this book.

We would like to thank especially all our colleagues at the Centre Hospitalier Spécialisé en Pneumologie in Chevilly-Larue : M. Angebault, D. Baud, J.-P. Bonniot, S. François-Coudray, M.-J. Postal and S. Roden for the help they have given us as well as M. Jondet, P. Le Pivert, A. Pecking, P. Renault and J.-P. Thiery.

We would also like to thank M. Mauriac and l'Agence Symbiose who produced the artwork for the illustrations and tables of this book as well as several posters that have been presented at various international congresses.

We would like to thank our colleagues and friends at the European Cryosurgery Group and the American College of Cryosurgery and hope that they will find in this book a justification of all their efforts to promote cryotherapy in each of their specialities for the benefit of their patients.

We would also like to thank Mrs Tanguy and Mrs Magor for all their hard work in producing the manuscripts for this book in spite of the authors.

To Nelly

To Stéphanie
Veronica
Vanessa
Matthew

List of authors

N.J. Bell, MBBS
Medical Advisor, The Medicine Group (UK) Ltd
General Practitioner, Oxford, England
Formerly Clinical Assistant British Hospital Paris and General Practitioner, Paris, France

J.-P. Bonniot, MD
Consultant, Centre Hospitalier Spécialisé en Pneumologie, Chevilly-Larue, France

J.-P. Homasson, MD-FCCP
Senior Consultant, Centre Hospitalier Spécialisé en Pneumologie, Chevilly-Larue, France

F. Lange, MD
University Lecturer, Hospital Practitioner in Pathology, Hôpital Henri Mondor, Créteil, France

Liu-Ping
Thoracic Surgeon, Shandong Cancer Hospital, Jinan, Shandong, The People's Republic of China

M.O. Maiwand, MD
Consultant thoracic surgeon, Thoracic and Cardiac Surgical Unit, Harefield Hospital, Harefield, Middlesex, England

G. Ozenne, MD-FCCP
Chest Physician, Centre Médico-Chirurgical du Cèdre, Bois-Guillaume, France

A. Pecking, MD
Consultant in Nuclear Medicine, Chef de service de Médecine Nucléaire, Centre René Huguenin, Saint-Cloud, France

B. Rubinsky
Professor of Biomedical Engineering, University of California, Berkeley, USA

J. Verdier
Engineer, Commissariat à l'Énergie Atomique, Centre d'Études Nucléaires, Grenoble, France

J.-M. Vergnon, MD
Chest Physician, Centre Hospitalo-Universitaire de Saint-Étienne et Unité de Recherche Biochimique de Pneumologie, Department of Medicine of Saint-Étienne, France

History of cryosurgery

Jean-Pierre Bonniot

The destruction of certain tumours by freezing is a relatively recent indication of cryotherapy dating from the end of the 19th century particularly if one considers that the effects of cold have been used in medicine for a very long time. The term « cryo » is actually used incorrectly in medicine as it really implies all temperatures below − 153° C when used in it's strictest sense in physics.

In 1862 Edwin Smith [1] discovered a papyrus of the 17th dynasty which was eventually published by the New York Historical Society in 1930. This papyrus written in red and black ink in 2 columns tells us that cold was used to treat infected wounds of the chest, fractures of the skull and various war wounds. In Homer's Iliad the beneficial effect of cold on war wounds is also mentioned.

In Aphorisms Hippocrates [2] describes how cold may be used in the treatment of haemorrhages and haematomas : « The cold eats wounds, it hardens the surrounding skin and causes a dull pain. It blackens (causes necrosis). Cold should be used in the following cases : 1) haemorrhages or to prevent them — it should not be applied directly to the bleeding part but to the surrounding area ; 2) all cases of inflammation where recent bleeding renders the area red and almost haemorrhagic (cold blackens old inflammation) ».

The cold was applied in the form of ice, snow or a mixture of various cooling agents. One can see from an Egyptian fresco of 3000 BC ice being produced by vaporization of water from a porous earthenware vessel ; in China in 1100 BC poets describe leaving buckets of water on the rooftop overnight where the temperature falls to below freezing. The Arab writer Ibn Abi Usaibia in 4th century described a cooling mixture using cold water and saltpetre (a mixture of sodium and potassium nitrate).

In the 11th century, Avicenne [3] (980-1037) produced a study of the anaesthetic properties of cold.

In the 16th century Severino in Naples used the effect of cold as an anaesthetic. The first major treatise concerning the use of cold in medicine was published in 1661 by T. Bartholini of Copenhagen [4] (« De Nivi Usu Medico ») and [5] (« De Figura Nivis Dissertatio ») using the aphorism of Hippocrates he identified the various possibilities on offer : « Nix est medicamentum, tum quia sale suo putredini adversantur, tum quia grata frigiditate extrema calidam viscerum interuperiem aestusque ; febriles qui pestilentiam plerumque ; comitantur et ebullitionem calidorum humorum antervertit, extinquit et inhibet. »

Following the suggestion of Hippocrate, the use of cold water in an acute gout attack was used with success on himself by W. Harvey [6] in 1650.

Baron D. Larrey [7] chief surgeon to the Imperial Guard of Napoleon described in his « Memoires of Military and Campaign Surgery » amputations of limbs carried out in Eylau during the Russian campaign without pain or haemorrhage following the application of snow and ice. This reflection by the famous surgeon is of interest as the effects of cold in surgery had been proposed after a detailed study of the effect of freezing on the body.

During the Russian campaign the external temperature fell to below − 50° C. « It is obvious that the effect of cold has a sedative effect on the brain and nervous system » ; some symptoms indicate freezing : « The part which is exposed to the cold is whiter than the rest of the body, all sensation is removed and the individual does not feel a sharp point. The fibres and capillary vessels become contracted and the fluids thicken and their circulation slows ». He also appreciated the importance of the speed of rewarming in the development and evolution of lesions. « The areas may remain in this state of asphyxia without dying and if the cold is diminished by degrees the equilibrium will easily be restored. If on the other hand the patients are suddenly changed from a frozen state to a warmer one where the temperature rises to a few degrees above zero then the areas blacken and gangrene is apparent. There is a sharp line of demarcation between the soft area and the healthy part, the scabs fall off at the ninth to thirteenth day. The loss of necrotic parts having taken place : the healing of the wound occurs rapidly and the patient recovers ».

Scientific research in physics and chemistry was progressing at the same time as that in medicine allowing cold to be achieved without using water. W. Cullen (1791-1867) between 1823 and 1845 liquified oxygen, nitrogen, carbon monoxide and dioxide, methane and hydrogen. The work of Carnot, Thomson and Joule in thermodynamics resulted in the invention of a refrigerator by compressing vapours to form liquids. The same Joule-Thompson effect (obtaining cold by a rapid release of a liquified gas from a capillary) is the basis of how some of the cryoprobes which are currently used for cryosurgery work.

For the first time in 1777 studies by J. Hunter [8] showed the destructive effect of cold and they were used in the treatment of tumours by J. Arnott [9-11] an English doctor from Brighton. In 1851 at the Universal Exhibition at Hyde Park in London he presented his « method of using cold as a therapeutic agent » using a mixture of ice and salt which allowed him to produce a local temperature of − 12° C. As an opponent of anaesthesia by chloroform inhalation he highlighted their harmful effects and he championed the local anaesthetic effect of cold, vaunting its efficacy and harmlessness. « I shall show by reports of cases of cancer treated by an anaesthetic temperature, that it furnishes us with a perfect means of relieving the pain of that dreadful disease, without producing the stupefaction and disturbance of the system which attends the use of narcotics ; and that instead of precipitating the unfortunate patient's fate, this congelation is not only calculated to prolong life for a protracted period, by arresting the accompanying inflammation, but may, probably, in the earlier stage of the disease and perhaps by destroying the vitality of the "cancer cell" exert a permanently curative action. »

These techniques were employed until the arrival of general anaesthesia and they were improved by B.W. Richardson [12] in 1866 who used the term « freezing » with ether spray. C. Redard [13] recommended ethyl chloride in 1891 as the temperatures achieved were even lower. This work was continued by J. and A.A. Arnott. J.H. Bennett from Edinburgh used the equipment of Arnott in 1849 to treat cancers with cold.

The vaporization of ether or ethyl chloride produced much lower temperatures than those achieved with previous cold agents such as ice and alcohol/ether mixtures. Other liquids appeared around this time such as liquid nitrogen and carbon dioxide. They were used for cutaneous lesions as indeed they are still used to this day. These liquid gases superseded all other methods because they were simpler to use and gave better results.

In 1871 J.F.A. Von Esmarch of Kiel published « The use of cold in surgery ». This was followed by a number of authors who published similar work, T. Bell in 1830, J.H. Bennes in 1849, T. Weedon-Cook in 1865 along with J.W. Bright who worked on the peripheral treatment of nerves.

Many authors published work using the effect of cold on tumours particularly in dermatology (C. Gerhardt 1885 used ice on cutaneous tuberculosis lesions) and gynaecology (Openchowski 1833 used ice cold water to treat chronic cervicitis).

According to L. Lortat Jacob [14] Lallier at l'Hôpital Saint-Louis in Paris was the first to use extreme cold as produced by methyl chloride to treat tumours in 1882. The temperatures reached with methyl chloride is around − 55° C but it is difficult to regulate the temperature. However if it is mixed with ethyl chloride it is a little easier to regulate.

In 1900, A.C. White [15, 16] started using liquid air. This agent was much better than anything that had been used before as more control could be exercised over the temperatures achieved by varying the pressure and the length of time of freezing. According to the length of treatment and the pressure, either a transient ischaemia could be achieved or else a complete freezing with secondary necrosis. The risks of explosion of the liquid air were diminished as demonstrated at a dermatology congress in Sarajevo in 1903 when liquid carbonic acid was used as a spray.

Pusey [17] from Chicago used carbon dioxide snow in 1905 by rapidly depressurising liquid carbonic acid. Carbon dioxide snow achieves a temperature of $-79°$ C. Liquid CO_2 at a pressure of 50 atmospheres may be kept easily in cylinders at a temperature of $15°$ C. It is very cheap because it is widely used in various industries. Pusey's method used sticks of carbon dioxide snow which were easy to use in dermatology. However they were very fragile as the slightest pressure would make them crumble. Another disadvantage of this method was the contamination of the area treated with germs. Several different cryocautery procedures were tried and Bordas in 1912 presented the first cryocautery to the Academy of Sciences. It consisted of « a silver tube of 1.5 cm cross section closed at one end by a flat surface of variable shapes. It is fixed in a double glass tube under vacuum and the end of the tube protrudes from the glass. The open end receives various cooling agents ». Research continued to produce a system fed directly with coolant but with a central regulator linked to a system to measure the pressure. In this way direct contact with the coolant was avoided and various cryogenic tips could be used instead.

The cryocauterer of Lortat-Jacob (Figs. 1, 2) [14] consists of a central metal tube about 18 cm long and 3 cm diameter. It is closed at the bottom with a piece of red leather of varying sizes.

A removable regulator is slid into the lumen of the tube. The innermost part of the apparatus is a white metal tube with the leather tip and regulator contained within it. The upper part of the wall has a scale with markings for 1 kg, 1.5 kg and 2 kg to measure the pressure of the apparatus applied to the lesion to be treated. The outer tube is of metal covered with a fibre insulation. A coil spring interposed between the two tubes allows the pressure exerted on the lesion to be measured. The cryocauterer is loaded manually with CO_2 gas mixed with acetone to make the cooling mixture.

In 1938, T. Fay [18-20] used freezing techniques in gynaecology for inoperable cancers to good effect by controlling pain, haemorrhage and tumour volume.

The observations of C. Geschichter and M. Copeland where bony metastases were more often found in the hottest parts of the body caused a renewed interest in localized cooling of the body. The effect of cooling the skin may produce a temperature 10-22° C below the core temperature. They used a capsule irrigated by continuous freezing water. After 5 weeks general and local improvement was noted. This technique has parallels with the treatment of inoperable cancers, lymphomas and glioblastomas with hypothermia.

H.L. Rosomoff and D.A. Holoday used the effects of cold in neurosurgery in 1954 following the work carried out in 1941 by L. Nins, C. Marschall and A. Neilson [21] where they looked at the effect of local freezing on the electrical activity of the cerebral cortex.

The development of more efficient instruments in 1959 by G.F. Rowbotham, A.L. Haigh and W.G. Leslie [22] who invented a fine cryoprobe

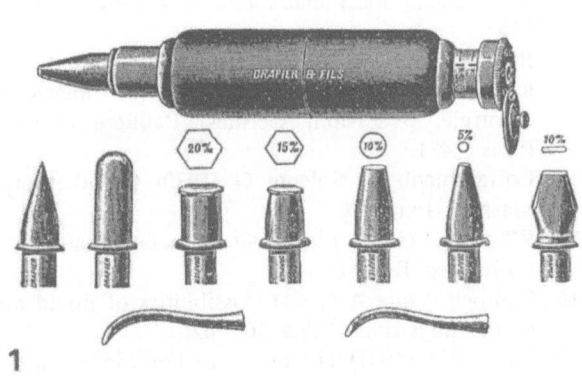

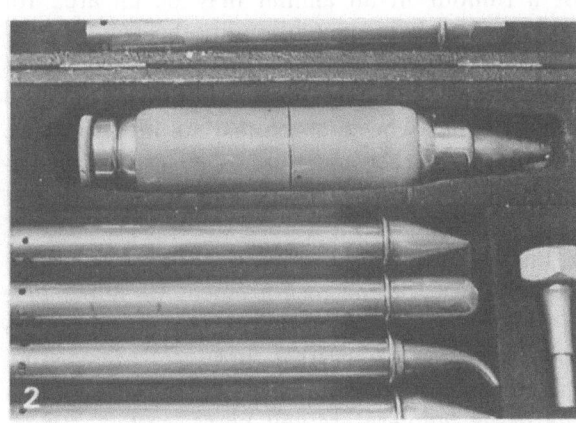

Figs. 1, 2. Cryocauterer of Lortat-Jacob

which could produce temperatures of − 20° C to destroy tumour tissue without harming surrounding healthy tissue led to modern cryosurgery. The tip of the cryoprobe which was driven by freon reached − 40° C. It was used for various applications ; destruction of deep tumours otherwise inoperable by conventional means ; ablation of vascular tumours by creating a barrier of frozen tissue around the tumour and various interventions such as cryopallidectomy and cryothalamotomy in extra pyramidal syndromes.

The recent rapid growth in cryosurgery is due to the use of liquid nitrogen as a cooling agent as first perfected by I.S. Cooper [23-30] and A. Lee. This apparatus works using the change of phase of a substance and consists of a cryoprobe with a metal tip where temperatures reach − 196° C. This was initially used to treat extra pyramidal disorders and intracranial lesions but it has also been used for treating rectal tumours, in ophthalmology and for the destruction of various other tumours.

In 1964 S.P. Amoils [31] improved the equipment by making probes for ophthalmic use which relied on the Joule-Thomson cooling effect. These probes worked with CO_2 and reached − 50° C. The technique was adapted by Rand [32-33] for transphenoidal hypophysectomy and for palliative treatment of various benign and malignant tumours by Cahan [34-36] which although not improving survival time, had a significant effect on pain and quality of life.

The possibility of an immune reaction to a tumour following cryoprostatectomy was studied by Ablin, Soanes and Gonder [37-40] who reported several regressions of metastases. The experiments of Myers, Hammond and Ketcham [41] showed that the transplantation of specific tumours after cryotherapy by chemical induction of a tumour in an animal may be an area for more research into cryoimmunotherapy.

The measurement of cryodestruction and its control have always been a problem and several methods have been developed to monitor this. The use of a thermocouple to measure the temperature of tissue surrounding a frozen area has been used — a temperature of − 15° − 20° C is known to be lethal to tissue. The measurement of resistance or the measurement of impedance (P. Le Pivert, 1975) [42-43], by the passage of a low frequency AC current through frozen tissue, means that for a resistance of 0.5 to 1 mega ohm the tissue temperature will be at least − 40° C. Thermography has also been used to estimate the area of freezing. The histological method of injecting fluorescein and recording the ultraviolet light is another method of visualizing the area of destruction. Conventional radiology, CT scans and ultrasound have also been used with varying degrees of success.

Due to their relative inaccessibility, endobronchial lesions and other cryosurgical techniques have only recently been introduced in chest medicine. The history of cryotherapy in chest medicine will be dealt with in another chapter.

References

1. Breasted JH (1930) The Edwin Smith Surgical Papyrus, vol. 3, University of Chicago Oriental Institute. Publication, Chicago : 217
2. Hippocrate (1532) Aphorismes par J.-F. Rabelais, Lyon
3. Avicenne (1498) Canonis Liber tertius
4. Bartholini T (1661) De nivis usu medico observationes variae. P. Haubold, Copenhagen
5. Bartholini T (1661) De figura nivis dissertatio. P. Haubold, Copenhagen
6. Aubery J (1949) Brief Lives, William Harvey, Scribner, New York : 231
7. Larrey DJ (1812) Mémoires de chirurgie militaire et campagne — Ed. F. Buisson, Paris
8. Barnard JDW (1980) The effects of extreme cold on sensory nerve. Ann R Coll Surg Engl 62 : 180-187
9. Arnott J (1845) On the present state of therapeutical inquiry. King, Brighton and Churchill, London
10. Arnott J (1851) On the treatment of cancer by the regulated application of an anaesthetic temperature. J Churchill, London
11. Arnott J (1855) On the treatment of cancer by congelation and an improve mode of pressure. J Churchill, London
12. Richardson BW (1866) On a new and ready mode of producing local anaesthesia. Med Times Gaz 1 : 115
13. Redard C (1891) Nouvelle méthode d'anesthésie locale par le chlorure d'éthyle. Congrès français de chirurgie. 5e session, Germer, Baillière et Cie, Paris : 431
14. Lortat-Jacob L, Solente G (1930) Cryotherapie, Masson, Paris : 6
15. White AC (1899) Liquid air in medicine and surgery. Med Rec 56 : 109
16. Cambell-White A (1901) Possibilities of liquid air to the physician. Jama 36 : 426
17. Pusey WA (1907) The use of carbon dioxide snow in the treatment of nevi and other lesions of the skin. Jama 49 : 456

18. Fay T (1940) Observations on prolonged human refrigeration. New York 40 : 1351

19. Fay T (1959) Experiences with refrigeration of the human brain. J Neurosurg 16 : 239

20. Fay T, Henney GC (1938) Correlation of body segmental temperature and its relation to the location of carcinomatous metastases : clinical observation and response to methods of refrigeration. Surg Gynecol Obstet 66 : 512

21. Nins LF, Marshall C, Neilson A (1941) Effect of local freezing on the electrical activity at the cerebral cortex. Yale J Biol Med 13 : 47

22. Rowbotham G, Haigh AC, Leslie WG (1959) Cooling canula for use in treatment of cerebral neoplasms. Lancet 1 : 12

23. Cooper IS, Lee A (1961) St J Cryothalamectomy-hypothermic congelation : a technical advance in basal ganglia surgery. Preliminary report. J Am Geriatr Soc 9 : 714

24. Cooper IS, Grisman F, Johnston PA (1962) A complete system for cryogenic surgery. St Barnabas Med Bull 1 : 11

25. Cooper IS, Grisman F, Gorek E, Williams R (1962) Cryogenic congelation and necrosis of cancer, a preliminary report. J Am Geriart Soc 10 : 289

26. Cooper IS, Stellar S (1963) Cryogenic freezing of brain tumours for excision or destruction in situ. J Neurosurg 20 : 921

27. Cooper IS (1963) Cryogenic surgery : a new method of destruction or extirpation of benign or malignant tissues. New Engl J Med 268 : 743-749

28. Cooper IS, Hirose T (1966) Application of cryogenic surgery to resection of parenchymal organs. New Engl J Med 274 : 15

29. Cooper IS (1969) Cryosurgery. Min Chir 24 : 1129

30. Cooper IS (1971) The present status of cryogenic surgery ID 10 : 34

31. Amoils SP, Walker AJ (1966) The thermal and mechanical factors involved in ocular cryosurgery. Proc R Soc Med 59 : 1056

32. Rand R.W. (1964) Stereotactic transphenoidal cryo-hypophysectomy. Preliminary report. Western J Surg 72 : 142

33. Rand RW, Dashe AM, Paglia DE, Conway LW, Solomon DH (1964) Stereotactic cryo-hypophysectomy 189 : 255

34. Cahan WG (1965) Cryosurgery of malignant and benign tumours. Fed. Proc. Fed. Am. Soc. Exp. Biol. 24 : 241

35. Cahan WG, Brockunier A (1967) Cryosurgery of the uterine cavity. Am J Obstet Gynecol 99 : 138-153

36. Cahan WG (1964) Cryosurgery of the uterus : description of technique and potential application. Amer J Obstet Gynec 88 : 410

37. Ablin RJ, Gonder MJ, Soanes WA (1969) Fluorescent studies of antibodies to male rabbit urogenital tissue. Experientia 25 : 994

38. Ablin RJ, Soanes WA, Bronson PM (1971) Auto antibodies to rabbit testis as a consequence of in situ freezing. Folia, Biologica Praha 17 : 429-431

39. Ablin RJ, Soanes WA, Gonder MJ (1971) Prospects for cryo immunotherapy in cases of metastasizing carcinoma of the prostate. Cryobiology 8 : 271-279

40. Ablin RJ, Sloane WA, Danaher J (1972) Immuno histologic studies of carcinoma of the prostate antibodies to prostatic tissues. Immunobiology 1 : 1425-1432

41. Myers RS, Hammond WG, Ketcham AS (1970) Cryosurgery of primate pancreas. Cancer 25 : 411-414

42. Le Pivert P, Binder P (1975) Utilisation des mesures d'impédance bioélectrique comme méthode de contrôle de la cryodestruction des tissus normaux ou pathologiques in vivo. CR Acad Sc Paris 281 : 1191-1194

43. Le Pivert P, Binder P, Ougier T (1977) Measurement of intratissue biolectrical low frequency impedance : a new method to predict per-operatively the destructive effect of cryosurgery. Cryobiology 14 : 245-250

The process of freezing and the mechanism of damage during cryosurgery

Boris Rubinsky

In recent years, the development of new techniques for genetically engineering macromolecules has generated hope that drug therapy for cancer will become available soon. However, this technique of therapy has not yet achieved its promised potential. Recent studies show that solid tumours are not easily accessible to macromolecules because of the particular pressure distribution in these tumours and the consequent fluid flow from the interior of the tumour to the exterior [1, 2]. Therefore, it appears that in the foreseeable future treatment of cancer will require extirpation of solid tumours coupled with chemical treatment of metastases and small tumours. Cryosurgery, which over the years has had great success in treatment of large solid tumours, may become even more important in the near future. New advances in the technology of imaging, such as intraoperative ultrasound, computer tomography and magnetic resonance imaging, have greatly increased the accuracy with which cryosurgery can be applied [3, 4]. Nevertheless, to efficiently combine cryosurgery and drug treatment with new genetically engineered macromolecules, it is imperative to understand the process of freezing and the mechanisms of damage caused by cryosurgery. This is particularly important if cryosurgery is to be accepted in today's scientific environment.

Tissue and biological organs consist of cells grouped in functional structures. The damage induced by freezing occurs at several levels, including the molecular level, the cellular level, structural level and the whole tissue. The mechanism of damage can be chemical or mechanical. During the last thirty years, the research on the process of freezing and the mechanism of damage during freezing has focused, in particular, on cells in suspensions. Much information is now available on this mode of freezing. Recently several studies have been initiated, aimed at understanding the process of freezing and the mechanism of damage at the molecular and structural level. This shift has occurred due to the need for a more fundamental understanding of the freezing processes and was made possible by the development of new experimental tools such as the low temperature electron microscopes, X-ray probes, magnetic resonance imaging as well as new numerical and analytical techniques for modelling freezing. The aim of this chapter is to briefly describe the information currently available on the general process of freezing in biological systems, at the cellular level and during freezing of tissue, and to describe new results on the particular process of freezing of solid tumours in the lung.

Freezing of cells in suspension

Cryosurgery which deals with the destruction of biological materials through freezing has developed in parallel with the area of cryopreservation, which deals with attempts to use freezing for the long term preservation of biological materials. Although the goals of these two areas are mutually exclusive, historically researchers in cryosurgery have explained the fundamental processes which occur during cryosurgery using information derived from research done on the use of freezing to preserve biological systems. The major event in cryopreservation was the serendipitous discovery that spermatozoa can survive freezing in the presence of various cryoprotectants, such as glycerol [5]. Since 1949 it was shown repeatedly that cells in a cellular suspension can survive freezing [6-10]. The use of freezing for preservation of cells has become routine, and is commonly utilized in many areas of medicine and biotechnology. Because of the wide range of applications much research has been done over the last four decades on cryopreservation of cells in solutions. In cryosurgery it has been generally thought that since organs and tissue are a composite of cells, the parameters which affect the freezing of cells in suspension will also similarly affect the freezing of cells in tissue. The effects of certain thermal parameters is well known. In this section these thermal parameters will be described first. This will be followed by a description of new results on the process of freezing of cells in suspensions. The new results lead to the conclusion that the thermal parameters which affect the viability of cells frozen in suspensions may be different from those which affect the viability of cells frozen in tissue.

The first decade and a half of research on the parameters which affect the viability of cells frozen in suspensions has led to the conclusion that « ... the temperature measurements most universally relevant to freezing injury in animal tissue was the rate of temperature fall (cooling rate, C/min) following the initiation of freezing » [11]. In general, the experiments which led to this conclusion were performed by freezing and thawing suspensions of cells, in vials, to different temperatures, with different cooling and

warming rates. After thawing, the viability of the frozen cells was determined using different tests such as evaluating the morphological integrity of the cells, trypan blue exclusion or the ability of the cells to continue to grow, in vitro. The results have shown that the plots correlating the viability of frozen cells to the cooling rates have the general « inverse U » shape, shown in a schematic form in Figure 1. Cells frozen with optimal cooling rates have the highest survival with survival decreasing from cells frozen with cooling rates higher and lower than the optimal. It was observed that the optimal cooling rate can vary between different types of cell by orders of magnitude. For example, it was observed that while in red blood cells the optimal cooling rate is of the order of 1000° C/min [9], in yeast the optimal cooling rate is 10° C/min, and in Hela cells the optimal cooling rate is 40° C/min [12]. Many of the experiments reported in the literature were performed with cells derived from cancerous tumours (i.e. the Hela cells). Therefore, it seemed reasonable to assume that if during cryosurgery cancerous cells in tissue are frozen with optimal cooling rates, they will survive freezing even at liquid nitrogen temperatures. Furthermore, different cells will survive the cryosurgical freezing protocol differently as a function of cell type and as a function of the overall thermal history which the cell experiences.

Together with the studies which led to the development of the viability curves discussed above, attempts were also made to establish a fundamental understanding of the thermophysical phenomena associated with the process of freezing in cells. The work has focused on developing mathematical models to describe the heat and mass transfer processes which occur during freezing of cells

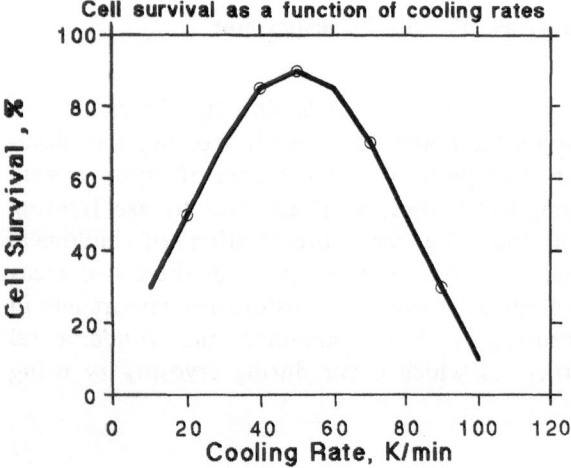

Fig. 1. Typical curve illustrates the « inverse U shaped » correlation between cooling rates during freezing and the viability of frozen cells. While the exact dependence of viability on cooling rates can vary between different cell types the general shape is usually the same

in suspensions, and on developing experimental techniques to observe the freezing of cells. Mazur has promoted the mathematical modelling of freezing processes in cells [13, 14], while Diller and Cravalho have contributed significantly to developing the techniques for studying experimentally the process of freezing in cellular suspensions [15, 16]. The results of the experimental studies and of the analytical studies show that the mechanism of damage during freezing can be explained through the heat and mass transfer processes which occur between the cells and their environment. The generally accepted explanation for the effect of cooling rates was proposed by Mazur [13, 14], who also developed the mathematical model for the process. Mazur suggested that during freezing of a cellular suspension the extracellular solution will freeze before the intracellular solution, because the extracellular solution has a larger volume and the probability for nucleation is a direct function of volume [17]. If the freezing occurs in a constant volume, since ice does not incorporate solutes, the concentration of saline in the remaining, unfrozen, extracellular solution will increase. Ice formation in the cell will depend on the probability of a critical ice-nucleus forming within the cell, which is an inverse function of the absolute temperature and a direct function of the volume of the cell [17]. For freezing with sufficiently low cooling rates, where the temperature is relatively high for long periods of time, the intracellular water can remain unfrozen while the extracellular solution freezes and becomes hypertonic. To equilibrate the difference in chemical potential between the intracellular solution and the extracellular solution water must leave the cell through the cell membrane, which is permeable to water but essentially impermeable to most of the solutes that are present.

Consequently the cell dehydrates and shrinks, and the intracellular concentration increases. It has been proposed originally by Lovelock [18], and developed by Mazur [19], that high electrolyte concentrations have a damaging effect, leading to the irreversible denaturation of intracellular proteins. The damage increases with the time of exposure. Because water transport is a rate-dependent process, freezing at higher cooling rates decreases the time during which a given cell is exposed to damaging conditions. This explains the increase in cell viability with an increase in cooling rates toward the optimum. However, when cells are frozen at supra-optimal cooling rates, the intracellular solution will become more thermodynamically supercooled, i.e. in a liquid state at a temperature lower than the phase transition temperature. This is a thermodynamically unstable situation which results in ice nucleation. Since higher cooling rates increase the supercooling the probability that intracellular ice will form increases with the cooling rates. Experimental evidence shows that the formation of intracellular ice is associated with mechanical damage to the cells, and this is assumed to be responsible for the decrease in cell viability at cooling rates above optimal [20]. Figures 2 and 3 were derived from analytical studies of the process of freezing in hepatocytes [21]. They show, respectively, the intracellular concentration, and the degree of intracellular supercooling, as a function of cell temperature during cooling with different cooling rates. From these figures it is obvious that at the same temperature, cells frozen with higher cooling rates will have a lower intracellular concentration and a higher degree of intracellular supercooling. These results are consistent with, and illustrate, the mechanism of freezing and damage discussed earlier.

Probably one of the most important research tools in cryobiology is the cryomicroscope [16], a device in which biological materials can be frozen with constant cooling rates on a special stage attached to a light microscope. The cryomicroscope is used to evaluate the change in the volume of cells during freezing and to observe the formation of intracellular ice. In general, the experimental results have verified the assumption that cells shrink when frozen with low cooling rates and that intracellular ice forms when cells are frozen with high cooling rates [20]. In the past, most of the cryomicroscopes were designed to generate a spatially uniform temperature distribution on the stage, which is cooled with constant cooling rate. However, recently Rubinsky and his coworkers [21-23] have suggested that the freezing process in large volumes cannot be accurately represented by a stage with a spatially uniform temperature distribution. In fact, during any freezing process, ice crystals form at a particular point and then propagate in the direction of the temperature gradients. Freezing does not occur uniformly, and is always a directional process, i.e. a process in which ice crystals propagate in a particular direction. Rubinsky has developed a new « directional solidification » cryomicroscope [23-25], which will be described in greater detail later in this chapter and which

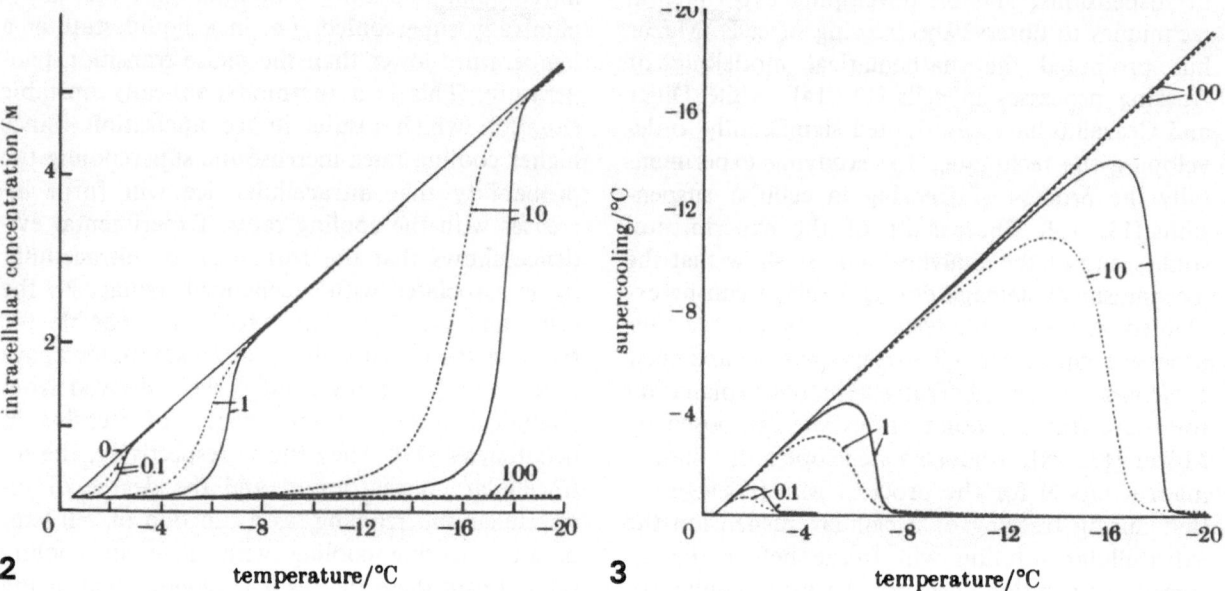

2   temperature/°C   **3**   temperature/°C

Fig. 2. Analytically derived values for the intracellular concentration in hepatocytes cooled with different cooling rates as a function of the hepatocyte temperature. The dashed line represents results of calculations performed for hepatocytes frozen in cellular suspensions and the straight line represents results of calculations performed for hepatocytes frozen in liver. Cooling rate (°C/min) as indicated (Reprinted with permission from Reference 21)

Fig. 3. Analytically derived values for intracellular supercooling in hepatocytes cooled with different cooling rates as a function of the hepatocyte temperature. The dashed line represents results of calculations performed for hepatocytes frozen in cellular suspensions and the straight line represents results of calculations performed for hepatocytes frozen in the liver. Cooling rate (°C/min as indicated) (Reprinted with permission from Reference 21)

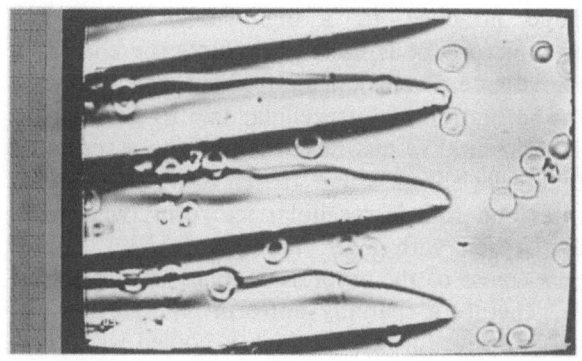

Fig. 4. Typical finger-like ice crystals form from left to right during freezing of saline solutions. Human red blood cells are seen between the ice crystals. The figure illustrates the observation that freezing processes of biological materials involve an interaction between ice crystals, the solution surrounding the ice crystals, and cells

more accurately simulates the directional process of freezing in large volumes of biological materials. Using this microscope it was shown that during freezing, ice crystals develop finger-like structures (see Fig. 4) with dimensions determined by such parameters as the velocity of propagation of the freezing interface and the spacial temperature gradients near the freezing interface. These parameters are only directly related to the cooling rate ; the produce of the velocity of the freezing interface and the spacial temperature gradient near the freezing interface is equal to the cool-

ing rate. During freezing of cells in suspensions, the cells interact with ice crystals. The physical phenomena which the cells experience are directly related to the particular interaction between the ice crystal structures, the solution surrounding the ice crystals and the cells (Fig. 4). Therefore, the cooling rates only indirectly describe the physical phenomena which occur during freezing of cells.

Recently, Rubinsky and De Vries [24], have shown that by modifying the structure of ice crystals it is possible to obtain, for exactly the same cooling rates, either complete survival of red blood cells or complete destruction of red blood cells. In a recent study, Beckmann et al. [26] have demonstrated that the viability of frozen lymphocytes cannot be correlated directly to the cooling rate. Their results show that the viability of lymphocytes frozen with identical cooling rates can vary for different combinations of freezing interface velocity and spacial temperature gradients. The viability does not depend directly on the cooling rate, which appears to be a thermal parameter of convenience with only an indirect physical significance. These observations may have important consequences for cryosurgery. They suggest that if the structure of the ice crystals which form during freezing of tissue is different from the structure of the ice crystals which form during freezing of cells in suspension, the viability of the cells frozen during cryosurgery will be different from the viability of cells frozen in solution with identical cooling rates. Therefore, the effects of cooling rates on cell viability determined from experiments with cells in suspension may not be relevant to the viability of cells frozen in tissue during cryosurgery, contrary to what many researchers, including this author, may have thought in the past.

Freezing of tissue

Cryosurgery is performed by applying a cooled probe to tissue and freezing the tissue from the tip of the probe in the direction of the temperature gradients which are established. Consequently, the frozen tissue will be exposed to different thermal histories, different cooling rates and different ranges of temperatures as a function of the distance from the tip of the probe. This combined with the inability to directly observe the process of freezing inside tissue, has made the study of the fundamental heat and mass transfer processes during cryosurgery extremely difficult. Faced with these problems, researchers in cryosurgery have drawn from the experience gained in studies with cells frozen in suspensions and have proposed similar criteria for damage to cells frozen in tissue as those found to affect the viability of cells frozen in suspensions, e.g. minimal temperatures of exposure or freezing with damaging cooling rates. In the absence of more accurate information, these criteria can provide useful guidance for cryosurgery. However, the recent

studies on freezing of cells in suspension, discussed in the previous section, suggest that the process of freezing in cells is not a simple function of cooling rates or minimal temperature of exposure. It appears that the process of freezing depends on the details of the interaction between ice crystals, the solution surrounding the ice crystals and the cells. It is quite obvious that the formation of ice crystals and the interaction of the ice crystals with the cells will be different during freezing of cells in solution and freezing of tissue during cryosurgery. Therefore, cells frozen in tissue will probably respond differently to the same thermal parameters from cells frozen in cellular suspensions.

Several researchers have studied the structure of tissue from whole organs frozen with constant cooling rates, microscopically [27, 28]. These experiments have shown that, in tissue, cells can freeze intracellularly or extracellularly as a function of cooling rates. Other studies in which the structure of tissue was observed after cryosurgery show that there is a very clear line of demarcation between tissue that was previously frozen and tissue that was not frozen [29]. Following cryosurgery, the cells in the frozen region have a disrupted structure, there was significant oedema in the frozen region and vascular stasis, with blood flow cessation in the small blood vessels of the tissue that was frozen [30]. Numerous experimental investigations show that one of the major sites of damage during cryosurgery is the vasculature, in particular the smaller blood vessels [31]. It has been stated by Le Pivert, in a review article on the basic aspect of freezing during cryosurgery [31], that « there is no doubt as to the preponderance of this mechanism (vascular damage) over the homogeneous destruction of the cryoinjured target, but the technical conditions to repeat and reproduce this thrombosis are poorly defined ». The second part of the statement by Le Pivert illustrates one of the major problems faced by researchers in cryosurgery, namely the difficulty in monitoring the thermal parameters during cryosurgery and in correlating the results of the surgical procedure to the heat and mass transfer phenomena which occur inside the tissue during cryosurgery.

The need for a better understanding of the heat and mass transfer processes which occur during freezing of tissue, the difficulties in controlling the temperature history during freezing of whole organs or during cryosurgery together with the difficulties in observing the process of freezing

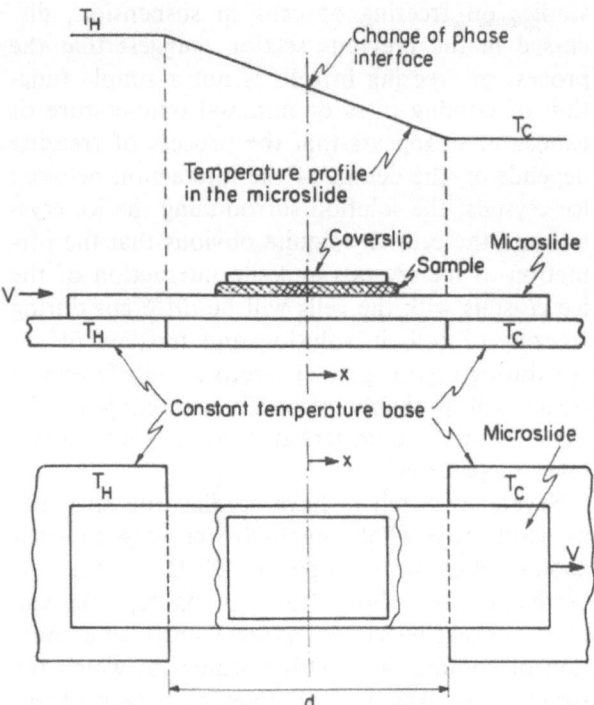

Fig. 5. Diagram of the directional solidification stage showing also the temperature distribution in the microslide

have led to the development of a new experimental technique to study this process. This technique uses the « directional solidification » cryomicroscope discussed earlier with respect to freezing of cells. The stage shown in a schematic form in Figure 5 consists of two constant temperature bases, separated by a gap. Each base can be maintained at a constant temperature, one base at a temperature above the freezing temperature and the other base at a temperature below the freezing temperature. A microslide rests on these bases. The system is designed in such a way that a linear temperature distribution is generated in the microslide between the high and the low temperature base. In typical experiments, thin slices of tissue can be placed on the microslide and moved with a constant velocity, across the bases. In this way the tissue slices, which take the temperature of the microslide can be frozen with constant cooling velocities between predetermined temperatures. After freezing, the tissue samples can be studied with a variety of microscopic techniques, including low temperature scanning electron microscopy and transmission electron microscopy, and the structure of the frozen tissue can be accurately correlated to the thermal history the samples have experienced.

Recent studies with liver slices frozen with a variety of cooling rates show that continuous ice crystals form in the blood vessels of the frozen tissue. The comparison of electron micrographs between normal and frozen liver reveal that in tissue frozen with low cooling rates there is a significant enlargement of the blood vessels containing ice, while the cells surrounding the frozen blood vessels shrink and dehydrate. This observation is illustrated by Figure 6. In tissue frozen with high cooling rates ice still forms in the blood vessels but the blood vessels are not expanded and the hepatocytes are frozen intracellularly (Fig. 7). A theory describing the mechanism of freezing was proposed based on these results [21]. Considering the probability for nucleation [17], ice will have a higher probability to form in the vasculature than in the cells of the tissue where the water is highly compartmentalized. Therefore, ice will begin to form and propagate through the vasculature, in the general direction of the temperature gradients but in the particular direction of the blood vessels. The water in cells surrounding the frozen blood vessel will remain supercooled. The solution in the blood vessels is isotonic and as the water comes out of the solution to form ice in the vascular system, the solutes in the remaining liquid will become more concentrated. To equilibrate the difference in concentration between the intracellular and vascular solution water will leave the cells surrounding the

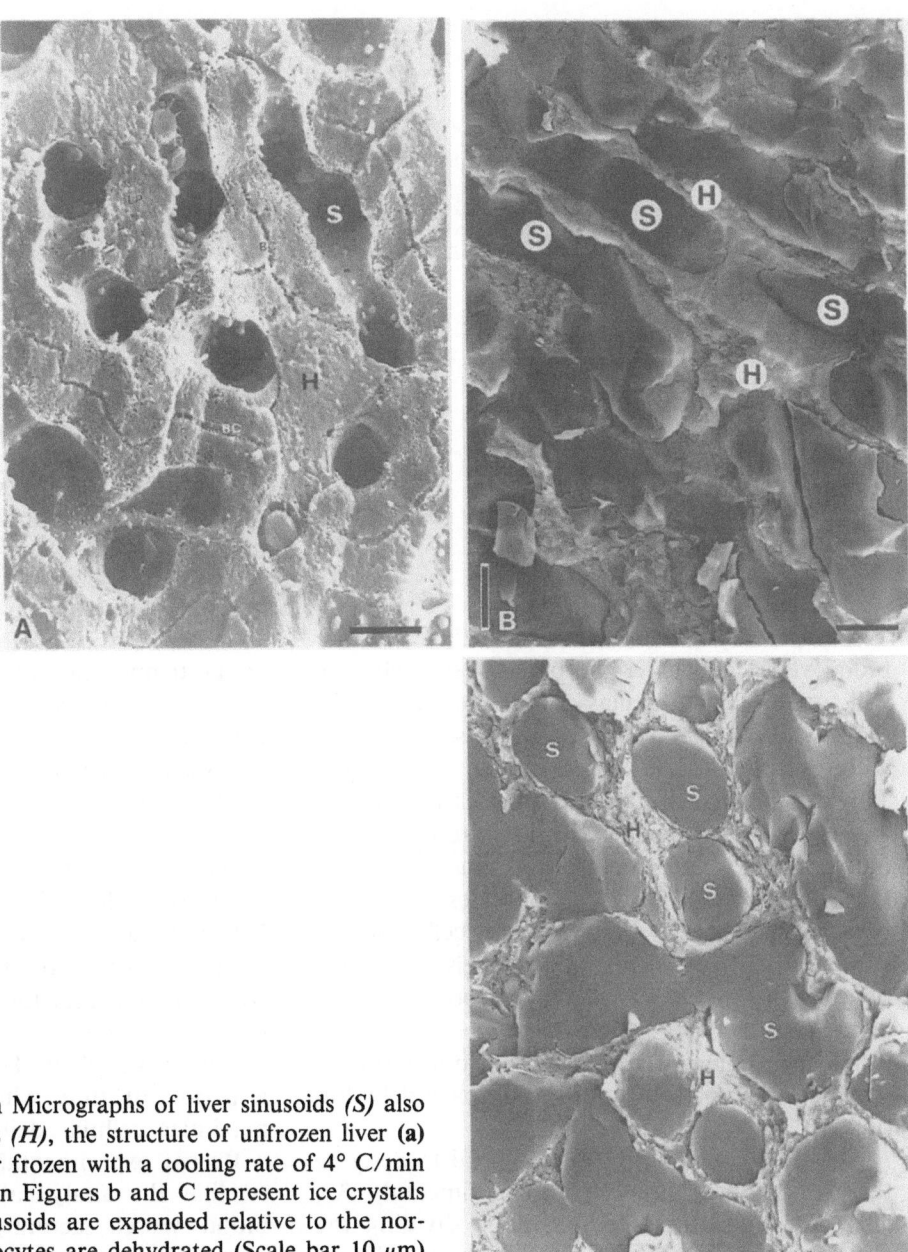

Fig. 6 a-c. Scanning Electron Micrographs of liver sinusoids *(S)* also showing adjacent hepatocytes *(H)*, the structure of unfrozen liver **(a)** is compared with that of liver frozen with a cooling rate of 4° C/min **(b, c)**. The smooth surfaces in Figures b and C represent ice crystals in sinusoids. The frozen sinusoids are expanded relative to the normal sinusoids and the hepatocytes are dehydrated (Scale bar 10 μm) (Reprinted by permission from Reference 21)

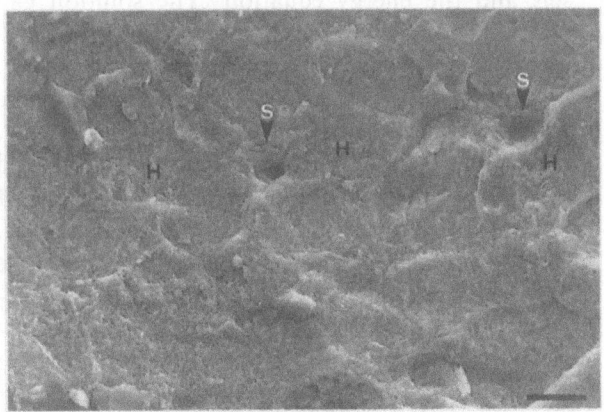

Fig. 7. Scanning Electron Micrographs of liver slices frozen with cooling rates on the order of 2000° C/min showing ice crystals in sinusoids (S) and small intracellular ice crystals in hepatocytes (H)

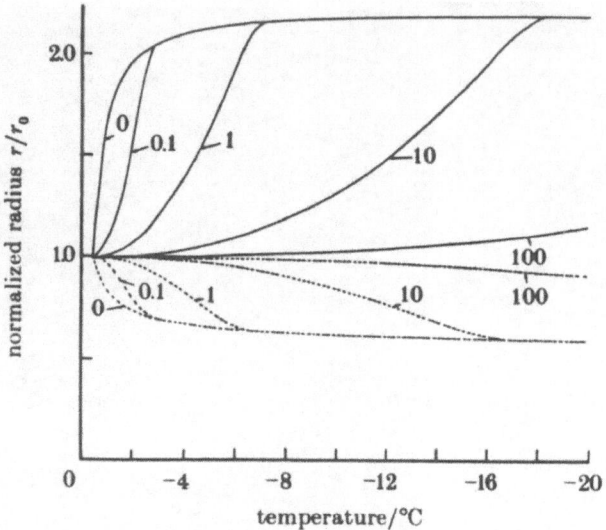

Fig. 8. Normalized radius of sinusoids (r/r_o), in liver frozen with different cooling rates as a function of temperature, showing the expansion of the blood vessels during freezing (straight line). Dashed line shows the shrinkage of the normalized radius of hepatocytes (r/r_o) during freezing with different cooling rates, showing the shrinkage of the hepatocytes (Reprinted with permission from Reference 21)

blood vessel and enter the blood vessel where it will freeze. Thus, the mass transfer of water into the blood vessel and its subsequent solidification will result in an expansion of the vasculature. This expansion will probably affect the structural integrity of the connective structure and of the blood vessels, which become non-functional upon thawing. Therefore low cooling rates will affect both the viability of the individual cells and the structural integrity of the blood vessels and of the tissue. During cooling with higher cooling rates, although ice will form first in the vasculature, the cells can become sufficiently supercooled for intracellular ice to form prior to complete dehydration.

New equations have been developed to describe the freezing process observed experimentaly [33, 34]. These equations are based on dividing the tissue into identical tissue units containing blood vessels and the adjacent cells, and solving for the mass transfer between the cells and the blood vessels and the energy equation. The solution can predict both the mass transfer and the temperature distribution during freezing of tissue. Figures 2 and 3, which were obtained using the equations derived in reference [21-33], show, respectively, the intracellular concentration and the intracellular supercooling during freezing of hepatocytes in liver, as a function of temperature, for freezing with different cooling rates. In these figures the intracellular concentration and the supercooling of hepatocytes frozen in cellular suspensions and in the liver are also compared. It is evident that the higher the cooling rate the low-

er the temperature at which the blood vessel will be completely expanded. For cooling rates of 0.1° C/min, the blood vessels will be completely expanded at a temperature of − 3° C, while for cooling rates of 10° C/min the complete expansion will occur only at temperatures as low as − 17° C. Since the expansion of blood vessels is likely to result in tissue damage it may be desirable to freeze slower during cryosurgery to obtain a better correlation between the extent of the frozen region and the necrotic tissue (Fig. 8). It may also be possible to achieve the expansion of the blood vessels by keeping the tissue frozen for a period of time which is sufficiently long to maximize cellular dehydration.

Recent experimental studies have demonstrated that the analytically predicted expansion of blood vessels actually occurs during cryosurgery [35]. In these studies the structure of tissue frozen during liver cryosurgery was examined with low temperature scanning electron microscopy. Tissue samples were taken at different distances from the tip of the cryosurgical probe. It was shown that near the cryosurgical probe, where the cooling rates are highest, the ice crystals form in the smaller blood vessels but the vessels have not expanded (Fig. 9). However, close to the outer edge of the frozen lesion the blood vessels containing ice have expanded and the adjacent cells have dehydrated (Fig. 10). It should be emphasized that the expansion of smaller blood vessels after cryosurgery was observed by other researchers as well [36, 37].

The recent experimental and analytical studies

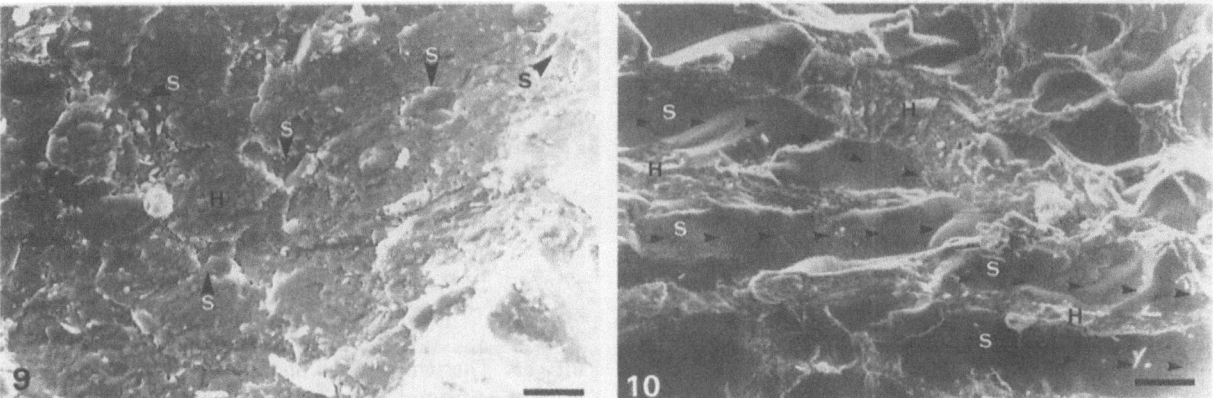

Fig. 9. Scanning Electron Micrograph of rat liver frozen during cryosurgery. The liver sample was taken from a region adjacent to the tip of the cryosurgical probe. Note the ice formation inside the sinusoids and intracellular ice in hepatocytes (Scale bar 10 μm) (Reprinted with permission from Reference 35)

Fig. 10. Scanning Electron Micrograph of rat liver during cryosurgery. The sample was taken from a region adjacent to the outer edge of the frozen lesion. Large continuous ice crystals are seen inside the sinusoids which are surrounded by dehydrated hepatocytes (Scale bar 10 μm) (Reprinted with permission from Reference 35)

discussed in this section, show that during cryosurgery cells will be damaged by mechanisms which are qualitatively similar to those which affect the viability of cells frozen in suspensions, i.e. the increase in intracellular concentration or the formation of intracellular ice. However, the quantitative effect of thermal parameters, such as cooling rates, will be different in cells frozen in tissue from that in identical cells frozen in cellular suspensions. Furthermore, an important mechanism of damage during cryosurgery appears to be the disruption of the structural integrity of the organ, in particular the disruption of the vasculature. This mode of damage may be dominant during cryosurgery and in the practical application of cryosurgery attempts should be made to enhance this mode of damage.

An analytical study of the process of freezing in the lung

The freezing process in tissue depends on the particular physiological structure of that tissue or organ. The lung is a special organ, characterized by a low macroscopic density. In the lung, solid tumours have a much higher density than the average density of the normal lung tissue. In this respect tumours in the lung are different from tumours in other organs. This is an important factor which will significantly affect the process of freezing in the lung. It has been recognized very early, that the average thermal properties of the lung are affected by the high air content of the lung [38]. The average thermal properties of the lung can be estimated using expressions for properties of composite materials described by Lunardini [39], where the thermal conductivity of the lung, k_l, is given by :

$$k_l = f_c k_c + f_a k_a \qquad (1)$$

Here, k_c and k_a are the thermal conductivities of cells and air respectively and f_c and f_a are the volume fraction of cells and air in the lung, respectively. The values for f_c and f_a are smaller than one and add to one.

The product of density and heat capacity in the lung, $(pc)_l$ are given by :

$$(pc)_l = f_c \cdot (pc)_c + f_a \cdot (pc)_a \qquad (2)$$

where the subscript c, stands for cells, and a, for air. Since in the lung only the cells will freeze, and not the air, the change in enthalpy during the freezing of an unit volume of lung tissue, L is given by :

$$L_l = f_c L_c \qquad (3)$$

In contrast to the lung, the solid tumours can be considered to be made only of cells with the appropriate thermal properties of cells. As a first approximation the thermal properties of the cells can be taken to be equivalent to those of water.

The process of freezing in a solid tumour surrounded by healthy lung tissue can be calculated using the thermal properties described above with

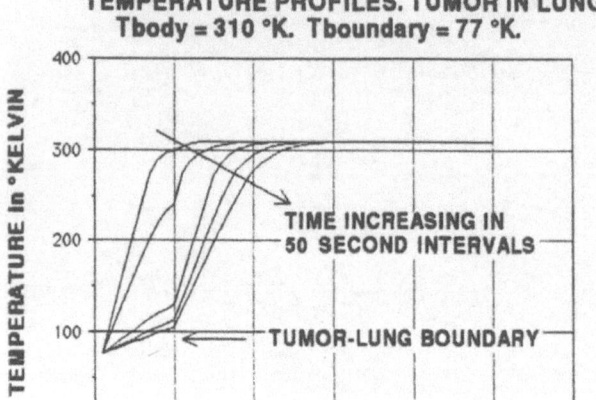

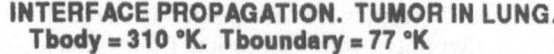

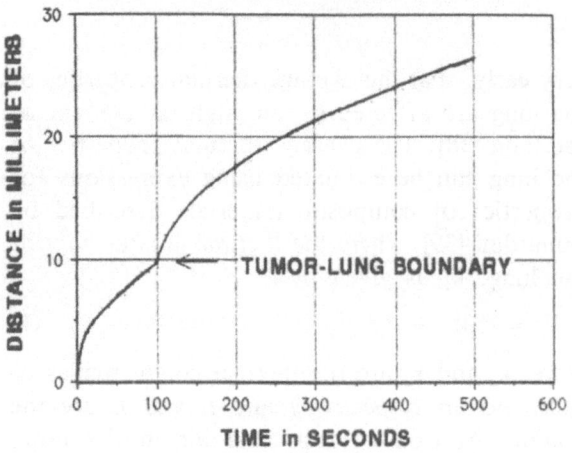

Fig. 11. The temperature distribution in a 10 mm solid tumour surrounded by healthy lung tissue frozen by cooling the outer surface of the tumour with a probe at liquid nitrogen temperature, 77K. The temperature profiles are given in 50 second time intervals [40]

Fig. 12. The distance of the freezing interface from the outer surface of the cryoprobe during the freezing of a 10 mm solid tumour surrounded by healthy tissue frozen by imposing on the outer surface of the tumour a temperature of 77K [40]

a variety of numerical schemes [39]. Using a finite difference scheme [39, 40], it is possible to predict the position of the freezing interface as a function of time as well as the temperature distribution during freezing. Applying this analysis to the freezing of a 10 mm solid tumour surrounded by healthy lung tissue, with a probe cooled by liquid nitrogen, generates very interesting results. The results described in Figures 11 and 12 show, respectively, the temperature distribution in the solid tumour and in the lung for different times after the onset of the freezing process, and the position of the freezing interface as a function of time. Figure 11 shows that the temperature distribution at the margin between the solid tumour and the normal lung tissue experiences a sudden discontinuity, after the solid tumour has frozen completely. When the normal lung tissue starts to freeze the temperature in the frozen solid

tumour suddenly drops to very low values. This behaviour can be explained by the fact that the energy required to freeze a certain volume of solid tumour is much smaller than the energy required to freeze the same volume of normal lung. This is evident from equation [3]. Consequently, once the whole solid tumour is frozen, since much less energy is required to freeze the adjacent healthy lung tissue, the cooling capability of the cryosurgical probe will go toward lowering the temperature of the frozen tumour. This behaviour may have important consequences in the application of cryosurgery to treatment of solid tumours in the lung. It provides an automatic mechanism for dropping the temperature of the frozen solid tumour to very low values by freezing slightly beyond the tumour into the healthy tissue. This may help ensure the complete destruction of solid tumours in the lung without the need for a special control mechanism. Nevertheless, the fact that much less energy must be removed to freeze healthy lung tissue may also have detrimental effects, as illustrated by Figure 12. Once the solid tumour is completely frozen the freezing of the healthy lung will require much less energy and the freezing interface will start accelerating in the healthy lung. The acceleration of the freezing interface once the solid tumour is completely frozen is evident from Figure 12. This suggests that, because of the special structure of the lung, it may be possible to accidentally injure a significant volume of healthy tissue if there is no appropriate control of the extent of freezing.

Future research

Significant efforts are currently being made to improve the clinical practice of cryosurgery. Impressive new advances are being made in techniques for controlling the process of freezing during cryosurgery using novel imaging techniques, such as intraoperative ultrasound, computer tomography and magnetic resonance imaging. With the recent clinical advances in the use of cryosurgery it is imperative to generate a much better understanding, both for the process of freezing and for the mechanism of damage during cryosurgery. There is no doubt that historically the field of cryosurgery has been dominated by clinical applications and has drawn its understanding of the physical processes from the work of researchers in the area of cryopreservation. Consequently, not much is known about the specific aspects of freezing during cryosurgery or the particular mechanisms of tissue damage during cryosurgery. Without this knowledge it is impossible to improve and optimize the procedure. The relation between the extent of the region frozen during cryosurgery and the region actually destroyed is not really known despite close to three decades of clinical application of « modern » cryosurgery. The issue of an immunological response following cryosurgery raised so many years ago by Ablin [41], was addressed only in an extremely limited number of studies, which have not yet led to any verifiable conclusions. There is no doubt that many more fundamental studies are needed on the process of freezing in tissue. The fundamental studies should be performed from the perspective of researchers interested in cryosurgery and not from the perspective of researchers working on cryopreservation of biological materials. A fundamental study on the process of freezing in different types of tumours, to elucidate the relation between the vascular structure of tumours and the freezing process would be extremely beneficial. The effect of the freezing process on the cancerous cell at a molecular level is an area with practically no research activity, despite the fact that it may hold the secret to the immunological aspect of cryosurgery. There is no doubt that cryosurgery has tremendous potential. To maximize this potential we must generate a more thorough fundamental understanding.

Acknowledgement. This work was supported by a grant from the Whitaker Foundation.

References

1. Jain RK, Baxter LT (1988) Mechanism of heterogeneous distribution of monoclonal antibodies and other macromolecules in tumors : Significance of elevated interstitial pressure. Cancer Research 48 : 7022-7032.
2. Jain RK (1987) Transport of molecules in the tumor interstition : a review. Cancer Research 47 : 3039-3051
3. Onik G, Rubinsky B (1988) Cryosurgery : new developments in understanding and techniques in low temperature biotechnology : emerging applications and engineering contributions. McGrath JJ Diller KR (Eds) pp. 57-80, Bed, vol. 10, Htd vol. 98, Asme Press, New York
4. Reiser M, Drukier AK, Feuerbach S (1983) The use of CT in monitoring cryosurgery. Eur J Radiol 3 (2) : 123-128
5. Polge C, Smith AU, Parkes AS (1949) Revival of spermatozoa after vitrification and dehydration at low temperatures. Nature 164 : 666
6. Smith AU (1950) Prevention of haemolysis during freezing and thawing of red blood cells. Lancet 250 : 910-911
7. Mollison PL, Slovitzer MA (1951) Successful transfusion of previously frozen human red cells. Lancet 261 : 862-864
8. Meryman MT (1966) Ed Cryobiology. Academic Press, London
9. Mazur P, Leibo SP, Farrant J, Chu HH, Hanna MG, Smith LM (1970) Interaction of cooling rate, warming rate and protective additives on the survival of frozen mammalian cells. The Frozen Cell J and A. Churchill, London
10. Luyet BJ (1949) Effects of ultra-rapid freezing and of slow freezing and thawing on mammalian erythrocytes. Biodynamics 6 : 217-230

11. Summary of the panel discussions, symposium on freezing rate (1966) Cryobiology 2 : 210

12. McGrath JJ, Cravalho EG, Huggins CE (1975) An experimental comparison of intracellular ice formation and freeze thaw survival of Hela S-3 cells. Cryobiology 12 : 540-550

13. Mazur P (1963) Kinetics of water loss from cells at sub zero temperatures and the likelihood of intracellular freezing. J Gen Physiol 47 : 347-369

14. Mazur P (1970) Cryobiology : the freezing of biological systems. Science 168 : 939-949

15. Diller KR, Cravalho EG (1971) An experimental study of freezing and thawing processes in biological cells. Cryobiology 7 : 191-199

16. Diller KR (1982) Quantitative low temperature optical microscopy of biological systems. J Microscopy 126 : 9-28

17. Turnbull D (1969) Under what conditions can a glass be formed ? Contemp Physics 10 : 473-488

18. Lovelock JE (1953) The mechanism of the protective action of glycerol against haemolysis by freezing and thawing. Biochem Biophys Acta 17 : 28-36

19. Mazur P (1977) Slow-freezing injury in mammalian cells. In : the freezing of mammalian embryos (Ed. Elliott K, Whelan J) (Ciba Foundation Symposium 52), Elsevier, Amsterdam : 19-42

20. Cravalho EC (1976) The application of cryogenics to the reversible storage of biomaterials in advances in cryogenic engineering. Timmerhaus KD, Weitzel DH (Eds) 21 : 399-417

21. Rubinsky B, Pegg DE (1988) A mathematical model for the freezing process in biological tissue. Proc R Soc London 234 : 343-358

22. Rubinsky B, Ikeda M (1985) A cryomicroscope using directional solidification for the controlled freezing of biological materials. Cryobiology 22 : 55-68

23. Chaw MW, Rubinsky B (1985) Cryomicroscopical observations on directional solidification in onion cells. Cryobiology 22 : 392-395

24. Rubinsky B (1985) Controlled freezing of biological materials using directional solidification. US Patent 453137 July

25. Rubinsky B, DeVries AL (1985) Effect of ice crystal habit on the viability of glycerol-protected red blood cells. Cryobiology 26 : 580

26. Beckman J, Körber C, Ran G, Hubel A, Cravalho EC (1990) Redefining cooling rate in terms of ice front velocity and thermal gradient : first evidence of relevance of freezing injury in lymphocytes. Cryobiology 27 : 279-287

27. Bank H (1973) Visualization of freezing damage, structural alteration during warming. Cryobiology 10 : 157-170

28. Hunt CJ, Taylor MJ, Pegg DE (1982) Freeze substitution and isothermal freeze-fixation studies to elucidate the pattern of ice formation in smooth muscle at 252K. J Microsc 125 : 177-186

29. Gilbert JC, Onik GM, Hoddick W, Rubinsky B (1985) Real time ultrasonic monitoring of hepatic cryosurgery. Cryobiology 22 : 319-330

30. Gage AA (1969) Cryosurgery for oral and pharyngeal carcinoma. A J Surg 118 : 669-672

31. Le Pivert PJ (1980) Basic considerations of the cryolesion. In : Handbook of Cryosurgery. Ablin, PJ (Ed) Marcel Dekker Inc., New York

32. Rubinsky B, Lee CY, Bastacky J, Hayes TL (1987) The mechanism of freezing in biological tissue : the liver. Cryo-Letters 8 : 320-381

33. Rubinsky B (1989) The energy equation for freezing of biological tissue. ASME Trans J of Heat Transfer 111 : 586-996

34. Rubinsky B, Eto TK (1989) Heat transfer during freezing of biological materials. Annual Review of Heat Transfer. Tien, CL (Ed) Hemisphere Pub. Co. New York 3 : 1-38

35. Rubinsky B, Lee CY, Bastacky J, Onik B (1990) The process of freezing and the mechanism of damage during hepatic cryosurgery. Cryobiology 27 : 85-97

36. Ninomiya T, Yosimura H, Mori M (1985) Identification of vascular system in experimental carcinoma for cryosurgery — historical observation of lectim VEA — 1 and alkaline phosphate activity in vascular endothelium. Cryobiology 33 : 331-335

37. Giampapa VC, Chanyul OH, Anfses AH (1981) The vascular effect of cold injury. Cryobiology 18 : 49-54

38. Staub NC, Storey WF (1967) Relation between morphological events in lung studied by rapid freezing. J Appl Physiol 17 : 381-390

39. Lunardini V (1981) Heat transfer in cold climates. Ch. 8, Van Nostrand, Reinhold, Co

40. Bischof J (1991) Experimental and analytical studies on the process of freezing in tissue. Ph. D. Thesis, Dept of Mechanical Engineering, University of California at Berkeley

41. Ablin RJ (1980) Ed Handbook of cryosurgery, Marcel Dekker, Inc. New York

The cryogens

Jacques Verdier

According to the literature [1-4] the core temperature needed for a lesion to be destroyed has to be between $-15°$ C to $-40°$ C, thus it is obvious that most cooling agents can be used as their saturation temperature is in the range of $-30°$ C to $-200°$ C as shown in Table 1.

This table gives the thermal properties of some of the more common fluids. They are generally used in the liquid phase so that on vaporization they remove heat at a constant temperature (heat of vaporization).

CFC's

The CFC's included in the table are commonly used in domestic and industrial refrigeration but they are rarely used for cooling in cryotherapy as it operates on an open circuit. In any case as a result of the destruction of the ozone layer they will be used less frequently in the future.

Carbon dioxide

Carbon dioxide (CO_2) seems to be an attractive proposition as it achieves a low temperature ($-79°$ C) and a high heat removal (574 kJ/kg), but unfortunately its expansion at atmospheric pressure produces carbon dioxide snow which is fine for direct application (as in dermatology for example) but it cannot be used in fine bore cryoprobes as the solid particles will block the flow of liquid in all but the largest probes.

Table 1. Thermal properties of cryogens

Cryogen		CFC_{12}	CFC_{22}	CO_2	CFC_{13}	N_2O	CFC_{14}	LN_2
Saturation temperature (atmospheric pressure)	°C	-30	-41	-79	-81	-89	-128	-196
Heat of vaporisation (at saturation temperature)	$kJ.kg^{-1}$	167	234	574	146	376	135	209
Vapour pressure at room temperature	10^5Pa	5,8	9,3	57,2	32,0	51,6	—	—
Critical pressure	10^5Pa	41,1	49,4	73,8	38,5	77,4	37,0	34,0
Critical temperature	°C	112	96	31,1	28,8	36,4	$-45,6$	-147

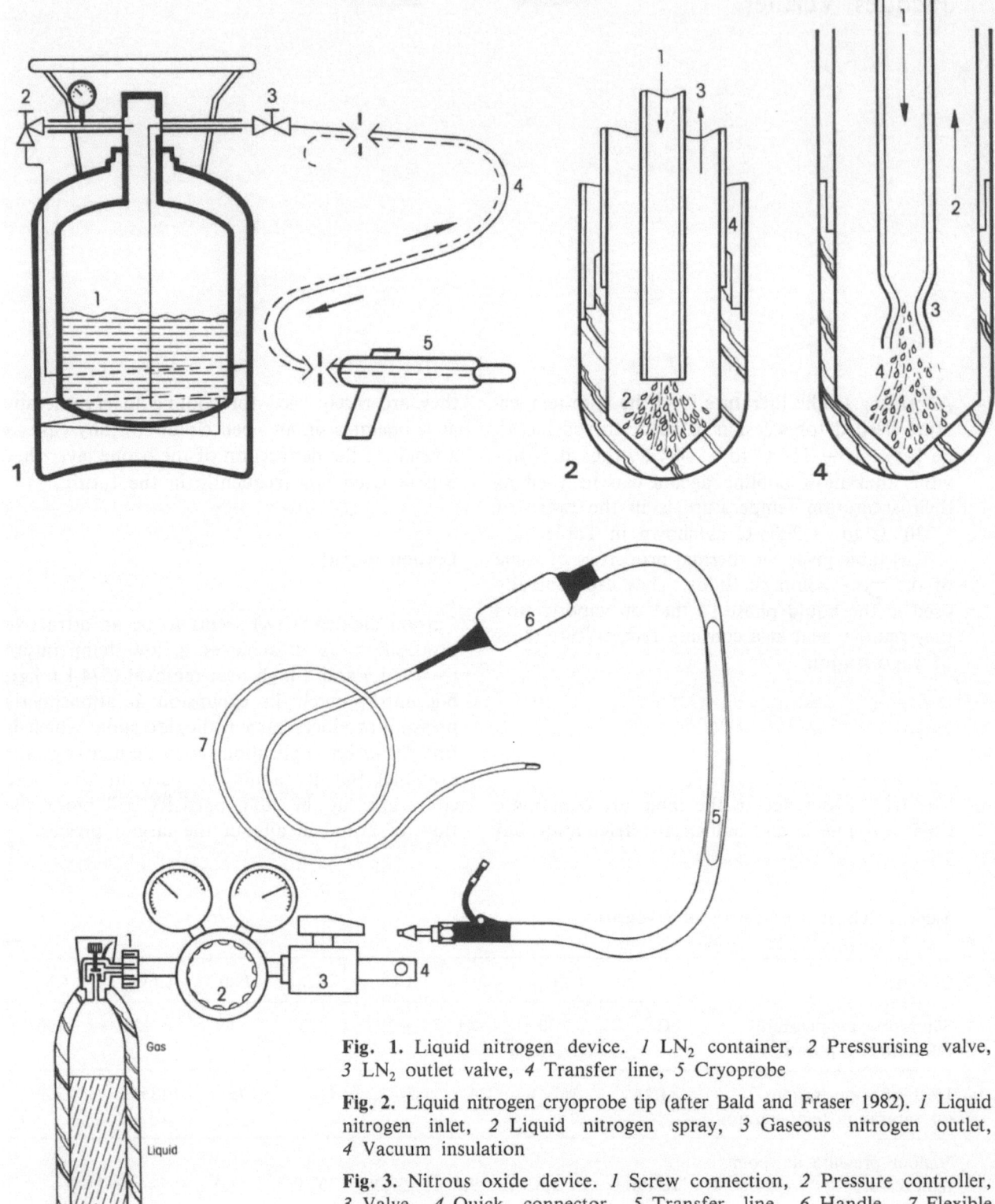

Fig. 1. Liquid nitrogen device. *1* LN$_2$ container, *2* Pressurising valve, *3* LN$_2$ outlet valve, *4* Transfer line, *5* Cryoprobe

Fig. 2. Liquid nitrogen cryoprobe tip (after Bald and Fraser 1982). *1* Liquid nitrogen inlet, *2* Liquid nitrogen spray, *3* Gaseous nitrogen outlet, *4* Vacuum insulation

Fig. 3. Nitrous oxide device. *1* Screw connection, *2* Pressure controller, *3* Valve, *4* Quick connector, *5* Transfer line, *6* Handle, *7* Flexible cryoprobe

Fig. 4. Nitrous oxide cryoprobe tip. *1* N$_2$0 (High pressure) inlet, *2* N$_2$0 (Atmospheric pressure) outlet, *3* Expansion nozzle, *4* Liquid N$_2$ spray

Liquid nitrogen and nitrous oxide

Nitrous oxide and liquid nitrogen are the two cryogens currently used for cooling cryoprobes used in destructive cryotherapy. They are both readily available in industrialized countries and they are not too expensive.

Liquid nitrogen is stored near its saturation temperature (− 196° C) in vacuum insulated containers in order to reduce the loss of liquid by evaporation. When the container is pressurized slightly the liquid can be transferred to a cryoprobe by a line placed at the bottom of the container. The flexibility of the transfer line is preserved by insulating it either by vacuum or a good thermal insulation.

When liquid nitrogen passes through the transfer line at room temperature initially it is evaporated so that gaseous nitrogen is in contact with the metal tip of the cryoprobe. This results in relatively slow cooling of the tip. When the temperature of the inner tube of the probe is sufficiently low to prevent evaporation of gas in transit, droplets of liquid nitrogen bombard the inner wall of the tip of the probe and they evaporate removing heat at a much quicker rate and producing very low temperatures (Fig. 2).

When the flow is stopped the amount of liquid remaining inside the transfer line must be evacuated via the cryoprobe thus thawing is delayed.

Many improvements have been made in order to make the transport of liquid N_2 easier, including the calefacient flow of liquid nitrogen (Leidenfrost), the electrical heating of cryoprobe tips and the use of heat exchanges in the probes [5-8].

Nitrous oxide

Nitrous oxide is stored at room temperature in high pressure bottles where the gas is in the liquid state. The pressure of the fluid inside the bottle is directly dependent on the temperature as shown in Table 2. Usually the vapour phase oc-

curs at the tip of the cryoprobe (Fig. 3) where it expands from a high pressure to atmospheric pressure (Fig. 4). This expansion lowers the temperature of the fluid and produces droplets of liquid in an equilibrium temperature at atmospheric pressure (− 89° C) see Table 1.

These droplets strike the metal tip of the probe and remove heat from the wall of the probe as they evaporate. The heat exchanges only occur in the distal one or two cms from the expansion nozzle between high pressure fluid coming in and low pressure gas exhausting. Thus the cooling power occurs just where it is needed, and in a very short time, as the metallic mass to be cooled is very small.

The transfer line and the cryoprobe are made of capillary tubes surrounded by sheaths of either metal or plastic depending on whether they are rigid or flexible. As they do not require any thermal insulation these cryoprobes lend themselves to endoscopic cryotherapy.

Table 2. Temperature — Pressure dependance of N_2O at saturation near room temperature

Temperature °C	0	5	10	15	20	25	30
Pressure 10^5Pa	30	35	40	45	50	56	63

References

1. Bald WB, Fraser J. (1982) Cryogenic Surgery. Rep Prog Phys 45 : 1384-1388
2. Le Pivert P, Binder P, Ougier T (1977) Measurement of intra tissue bioelectrical low frequency impedance : a new method to predict per-operatively the destructive effect of cryosurgery. Cryobiology 14 : 245-250
3. Gage AA (1979) What temperature is lethal for cells. J Derm Surg Oncol 464 : 453-460
4. Ablin RJ (1980) Handbook of Cryosurgery. M. Dekker — Inc. New York 17-20 and 89-94
5. Orpwood RD (1981) Biophysical and engineering aspects of cryosurgery. Phys Med Biol 26 : 567-569
6. Tian BT, Zhang GG (1981) A new type of medical liquid nitrogen cryogenic apparatus. In : Cryosurgery and medical applications of refrigerations ; current situation and perspectives. IIR Comm. C_1, Warsaw 3 : 131-134
7. Bald WB, Fraser J (1982) Cryogenic surgery. Rep Prog Phys 45 : 1419-1428
8. Gravil B, Sauvigné G, Verdier J, Lacaze A, Le Pivert P (1981) Sonde cryochirurgicale autorégulée et flexible. In : Cryosurgery and medical applications of refrigeration : current situation and perspectives. IIR ; Comm C_1, Warsaw 3 : 123-129

Monitoring techniques

Jacques Verdier

It is essential to predict and control the area of necrosis which will occur following freezing of a tissue. The necrosis occurs within the volume of the « ice ball » which forms around the tip of a cryoprobe. This ice ball may be monitored by direct vision or else by measuring some physical parameter such as temperature or electrical conductivity.

It is thought that freezing is most lethal when the eutectic freezing point has been reached for a tissue and thus a measurement of the eutectic spatial extension of an ice ball will correspond to the area of tissue damage.

Thermal methods

Thermocouple needles may be inserted into a tissue and located at appropriate places to mark the limit where a desired temperature has to be reached [1]. Continuous recording of several thermocouples inserted in and around a lesion will provide useful information concerning :
- the rate of cooling,
- the time of freezing,
- the rate of thawing.

The temperature of eutectic freezing may be determined for different tissues depending on their chemical composition [2] but it requires the insertion of several needles and still relies on good clinical judgement and experience to interpret the results [3].

Temperature sensor technology has made great advances lately and the development of fibre optic needles for spectral analysis of thermal emission may be applied to cryotherapy in the near future. Other thermal methods such as infra red thermography [4] and heat flux mapping [5] have been described in the literature but they are only of scientific interest as they cannot be applied to endoscopic cryotherapy due to the restricted access.

Volumetric methods

The volume of the ice ball formed may be accurately assessed by various conventional methods of measuring changes in physical structure such as ultrasonography or x-ray tomography but the extent of eutectic freezing is not possible to measure in this way. Although ultrasonography is easier to use neither method has been applied to clinical cryotherapy with much success.

Electrical methods

When a tissue freezes its resistance changes markedly and the best way of measuring this is to use AC in the range of kilohertz frequencies [6]. The electrical capacitance of the tissue is connected in parallel with its resistance so that total impedance is measured.

Le Pivert [7] developed this method in 1974 by using electrode needles inserted in and around the lesion to be destroyed in similar fashion to the thermocouple method described above.

When freezing occurs in tissue the impedance

measured between two electrodes jumps from a level of 0.5 kΩ in the unfrozen state to anything between 10 to 50 kΩ as more and more pure water ice crystals form and the electrolyte remain-

ing becomes more concentrated. A second, more rapid rise in impedance occurs as the eutectic temperature is reached and the electrolyte freezes in a flash — the impedance at this state is some-

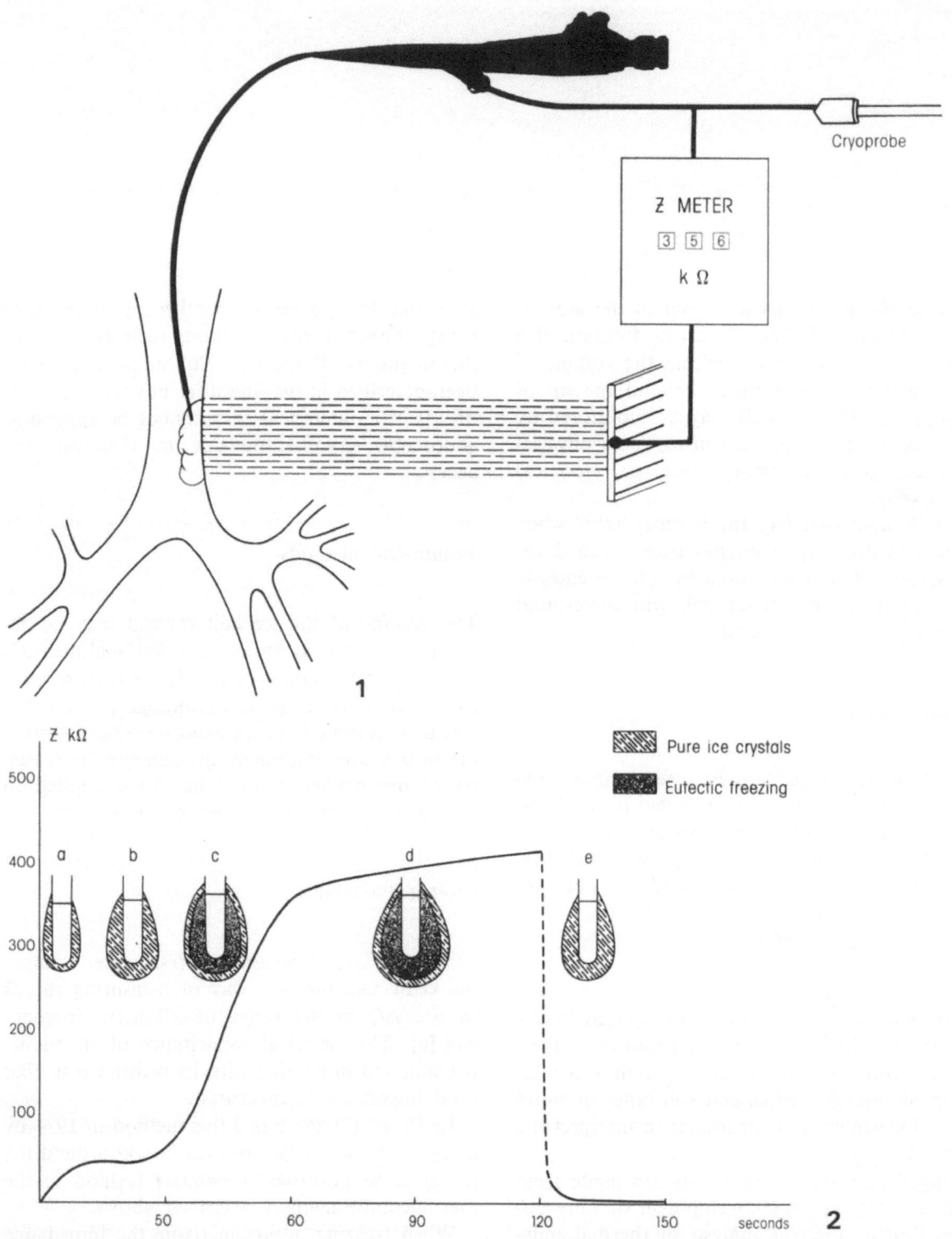

Fig. 1. Method of measuring the impedance using the cryoprobe as an electrode

Fig. 2. Typical time variation of the impedance and correlated increase of the eutectic area within the ice ball

where between 500 to 1000 kΩ. If the electrodes are well placed the area of eutectic freezing may be monitored and controlled.

This impedance metric method has been adapted for use in endoscopic cryotherapy without resorting to multiple needle insertion to map the frozen area. It works by employing the metal tip of the cryoprobe as an impedancemetric electrode — a metal pad placed on the skin of the patient acts as the other electrode (Fig. 1).

As described above the increased impedance correlates with the freezing of tissue. Figure 2 demonstrates a typical fluctuation of impedance during a session of cryotherapy.

These changes in impedance may be explained by the following observations made when a cryoprobe is plugged into physiological saline (0.9 % NaCI). Before use the impedance measures less than 1 kΩ. As soon as the N_2O starts to flow a thin layer of ice forms, coating the tip of the cryoprobe — this corresponds to an initial rise of impedance to 10 kΩ. The impedance continues to rise and stabilizes around 50 kΩ. During this phase ice crystals are continuing to form around the tip of the cryoprobe but a small amount of concentrated saline remains between the crystals.

After a further 15 to 40 seconds there is a further sharp rise in impedance at the rate of $dz/dr \geqslant 15$ kΩ/s^{-1} to between 200 to 500 kΩ (usually 400 kΩ) which corresponds to the eutectic freezing of all liquids between the tip of the probe and the freezing border.

At this point a steady state is reached which lasts for 1 to 2 minutes during which time the impedance and the ice ball volume remain constant. The ice ball is in two parts, an inner solid core where eutectic freezing has occurred surrounded by a layer of ice crystals mixed with concentrated saline solution.

When the flow of N_2O is stopped the ice ball melts comparatively slowly (about 30 seconds) although the drop in impedance only takes a few seconds.

This is because the eutectic part of the ice ball which only occupies a small percentage of the total ice ball melts at $-21°$ C as against $0°$ C.

Although the events described above are those that occur with normal saline, and living tissue is more complex, it serves as a good model to explain the impedance changes encountered when tissue is frozen with a cryoprobe. This system of monitoring is used with both the rigid and flexible cryoprobes which are manufactured in France.

References

1. Bald WB, Fraser J (1982) Cryogenic surgery. Rep Prog Phys 45 : 1426-1428
2. Lacaze A, Le Pivert P, Verdier J (1987) Le froid en chirurgie. Hermann Ed. Paris 56-57
3. Le Pivert P (1980) Basic considerations of the cryolesion. In : Handbook of cryosurgery. Ablin RS, Dekker M, Inc. New York : 42-58
4. Bradley PF (1977) Thermography as an aid to cryosurgery. Acta Thermogr 2 : 83
5. Harly S, Aastrup JE, Elbrondond O (1977) Heat flux measurement during cryosurgery. Cryobiology 14 : 609-613
6. Le Pivert P, Binder P (1975) Utilisation des mesures d'impédance bioélectriques comme méthode de contrôle de la cryo-obstruction « in vivo ». C R Acad Sc Paris 285 : 1191-1194
7. Le Pivert P (1974) Cryochirurgie en cancérologie « Contribution expérimentale à l'étude de la cryo-destruction des cellules tumorales in vivo » (Thesis), Lyon University

History of tracheo-bronchial cryotherapy

Jean-Paul Homasson

The use of cryosurgery in chest medicine is relatively recent compared to other medical specialties such as dermatology, ENT, maxillo-facial surgery [1], etc. where the lesions are easily accessible. In fact chest medicine is reliant on endoscopes with a very narrow bore in order to treat any tracheal or bronchial lesions. The cryoprobes must be of a sufficiently narrow diameter in order to pass through the lumen of rigid or fibre optic bronchoscopes.

After an initial experimental interest in the technique carried out in the United States between 1975 and 1982 it was dropped in favour of the laser.

In 1986 workers in France and Great Britain started to use and develop the technique again and since then it is being used more frequently. At present it is used in Spain, Portugal, Italy, Czechoslovakia and Belgium and its use is likely to spread throughout Europe and eventually the USA. It is soon to be introduced in Asia and undoubtedly Africa in the near future.

Experimental studies

Following initial work by Gage [2] who described the regrowth of bone following freezing and by Grana [3] who published his experiences of cryosurgery in the trachea of healthy dogs, Thomford [4] carried out a study describing the morphological changes in canine trachea after freezing. The aim of this work was to demonstrate the use of cryosurgery on tracheal tumours without causing perforation. A cryoprobe was applied to the external surface of the trachea which was frozen via a thoracotomy under general anaesthetic. The area treated was observed endoscopically on the 1st, 3rd and 7th day and then weekly following cryotherapy. Biopsies were taken after five minutes, 2 hours, 6 hours, 24 hours and then 3 days and weekly thereafter.

After an initial phase of hyperaemia and oedema the mucous membrane returned to normal over seven days. Serial biopsies charted the different stages of the lesion. Five minutes after freezing there was interstitial oedema and distortion of the cell membranes but there was no change in the cartilage. The time of maximum cryodestruction was 24 hours after cryotherapy with marked changes to the mucosa and destruction of submucosal glands combined with an inflammatory infiltration. There was a widespread vascular thrombosis and the perichondrium was thickened with an absence of chondrocytes. From the 72nd hour onwards there was a gradual re-epithelialisation, the oedema disappeared and new cartilage was formed with chondrocytes around the edge of the lesion. By the 5th week chondrocytes were present throughout the cartilage but there were still no ciliated cells. However the freezing did not lead to perforation or fibrosis, the cartilage returned to normal and it was only the ciliated cells which did not reappear.

Following this basic study the same team [5] studied the effect of cryotherapy on tracheal tumours in rats. Wistar rats were surgically prepared by implanting a 1 mm cube of Walker 256 carcino sarcoma between the thyroid isthmus and the trachea. After the tumour had invaded the trachea, freezing was accomplished by applying the tip of the probe to the tumour mass for a period of 15 sec. After thawing, the procedure was repeated until the total period of freezing equalled two minutes. Necropsy studies demonstrated complete eradication of tumour without permanently altering the gross architecture of the trachea. In conclusion, cryotherapy may be of vallue in the management of selected patients with neoplasms of the trachea.

Neel and colleagues (Mayo Clinic and Mayo Foundation, Rochester, Minn) published a similar study to Thomford. They studied the effect of a complete circumferential cryonecrosis induced in the trachea of 8 mongrel dogs, and also the effect of endoscopic freezing of the trachea in a further 3 dogs [6]. In the first study the trachea was exposed surgically using a median cervical incision and 5 or 6 rings were frozen, producing a cryonecrotic lesion over 15-18 mm of trachea. In the second series of 3 dogs they underwent bronchoscopy and a 6 mm diameter cryoprobe was passed. Several areas were frozen, namely the trachea anteriorly and posteriorly, the carina and main bronchi in several places. Repeat control bronchoscopies were carried out on the 1st, 4th, 7th, 14th and 28th day following freezing. All the dogs survived and had fully recovered 12 hours after the anaesthetic. One dog suffered a vocal cord paralysis due to freezing of the recurrent nerve but this resolved after one week. Thus the action of freezing the trachea was well tolerated. Twenty-four hours after freezing there was some oedema to the area and a slight ulceration was also noted on bronchoscopy. This was followed by localised necrosis and rapid regeneration of the mucosa. The trachea was not distorted and by the end of the first week the mucosal surface had regenerated with cuboidal epithelium. The cartilage was unchanged but there were increased numbers of chondrocytes in the adjacent areas. The histological appearances were the same whether the freezing was produced externally to the exposed trachea or else endoscopically using a cryoprobe. There was complete mucosal recovery after 4 weeks.

Following this the same workers [7] studied the effect of freezing on lung tissue in ten animals by thoracotomy and multiple applications of a cryoprobe. The lesions produced were very similar to an acute haemorrhagic infarct with complete collapse and a fibrosis of the surrounding pulmonary tissue with several areas of haemorrhagic necrosis.

Gorenstein and his team at the Mayo Clinic [8] published a study where endoscopic cryotherapy was applied to 24 healthy dogs. The freezing process was controlled using internal thermocouples, and various points in the tracheo-bronchial tree were frozen (carina, main bronchi and superior lobe bronchi). Thirteen dogs also underwent pulmonary freezing through the bronchus. The results of this study confirmed those obtained by Neel.

Carpenter et al [9] repeated the same study in 20 healthy mongrel dogs. The study was done in two parts. Eight dogs of a first group were anaesthetized and a right thoracotomy was performed to expose the right upper lobe bronchus ; external freezing of the bronchial serosal surface was accomplished by using a closed tip Frigitronics cryoprobe 15 mm in diameter. The temperature of the probe's tip was maintained at − 160° C to − 170° C, and three freezing cycles of two minutes each were used in each location. Monitoring of the temperature of the target area and peripheral tissue was carried out with thermocouple needles. A right thoracotomy approach was used to expose the right upper lobe bronchus of twelve other mongrel dogs ; a longitudinal bronchotomy was performed permitting good exposure of the bronchial lumen and the three peripheral divisions of the right upper lobe bronchus. In eight of these dogs, a cryoprobe 6 mm in diameter was introduced through the bronchotomy. Each peripheral bronchus including the site of bronchotomy was frozen three times (temperature maintained at − 160° C to − 170° C). In four control dogs an identical procedure excluding the cryosurgery was performed. 180 days after cryosurgery, bronchograms were carried out in five dogs. All dogs survived the procedures and remained in good health throughout the follow-up period of six months. After external bronchial (serosal) freezing, the serosal and mucosal surfaces of the bronchus were hyperaemic and well demarcated from normal tissue. There was minimal edema. Fourteen days after freezing, the bronchus appeared normal, both at the serosal and mucosal surfaces.

In the animals that had bronchotomies but no cryosurgery (controls), no evidence of disruption of the bronchotomy incision was noted. After cryosurgery, gross changes paralleled those stated previously. Rapid healing of the bronchotomy incision occurred in all animals, and by one month following freezing, all tissue appeared normal ; there was no evidence of formation of a

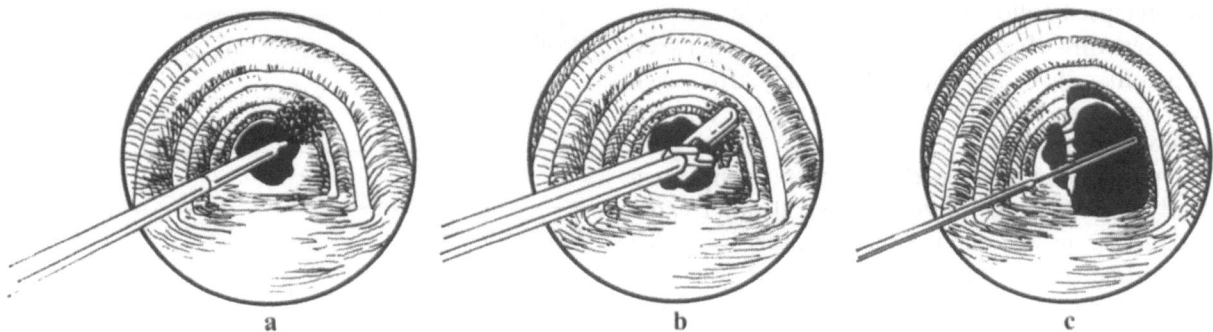

a   b   c

Fig. 1. Endoscopic cryoresection technique. a Application of cryoprobe to an area of fibrous stricture in the mid portion of the trachea. A relatively localized area of tissue is frozen due to rapid temperature dissipation. b Endotracheal resection of frozen tissue using standard angled biopsy forceps. c Following repeated cryoresection of 180 degrees of the tracheal circumference, the area was injected with submucosal corticosteroid (after Journal of Paediatric Surgery, 1978)

stricture or other alteration in architecture or function. Microscopic studies were made 1, 4, 7, 14, 30 and 180 days after cryosurgery. Shortly after the procedure, complete necrosis of the mucosa was evident in the cryolesion and no glandular structures were present. The submucosa was oedematous, with extensive thrombosis of vessels. The cryolesion extended to the full thickness of the wall and in the bronchotomy specimen encompassed the incision. The framework of the bronchus remained intact. Fourteen days after cryosurgery, cuboidal epithelium was seen in many areas of the target site. Cartilage was intact, but many of the nuclei were pyknotic. Thirty days after cryosurgery, cuboidal epithelium covered the central target and normal ciliated columnar epithelium was seen in some areas. Thrombi still remained in many vessels. Cartilage in the target area was devoid of normal nuclei. The bronchotomy was closed and filled with fibrous tissue. Sixty to 180 days after cryosurgery, there was continuous ciliated epithelium over the target area. Several areas of new cartilage were apparent alongside original cartilage that had lost viable nuclei.

Bronchograms carried out six months after external bronchial freezing and after combined bronchotomy and cryosurgery demonstrated normal clearance of dye. There was no evidence of stricture formation. Contrast material cleared quickly and could not be seen five days after instillation.

This study was of great interest and opened the door to the use of cryosurgery in humans. The destructive power of cold had been confirmed but the healing of the trachea and bronchi was good

with restoration of normal ciliated epithelium without any stenosis or shrinkage and with minimal oedematous reactions. No perforation had occurred.

Carpenter et al. [10] compared endoscopic cryosurgery and electrocoagulation of bronchi and found that electrocoagulation failed to completely destroy mucosa and glands. Skip areas of normal tissue were commonly observed. Architectural support was lost because cartilage was destroyed, and this led to collapse of the bronchial wall and to formation of a stricture. In contrast endoscopic cryosurgery produced a uniform and predictable lesion, with regrowth of normal respiratory mucosa.

Endobronchial cryosurgery in man

The first case was published in 1968 [11]. The patient had a carcinomatous obstruction of a bronchus with infection in the distal lung area. Endobronchial freezing, using a 5 mm cryoprobe (Manufactured by Linde Division, Union Carbide Corporation, 270 Park Avenue, New York, New York 10017) through a bronchoscope, achieved improved aeration of the lung behind the obstruction so that the patient was able to go home. This benefit was only temporary. The patient was treated on 5 additional occasions, 2-3 months apart, in order to maintain the airway. He died 16 months later from the cancer.

In 1975, another case was reported [12]. It consisted of a man suffering from an infiltrating bronchial carcinoma situated at the carina who had relapsed following radiotherapy. He received five sessions of endoscopic cryotherapy between September 1973 and April 1974 and after each session his respiratory function improved and the tumour regressed.

At the same time as they were working on a study with 24 dogs Gorenstein et al. [8] treated 6 patients using endoscopic cryosurgery. The cryoprobe which measured 6 mm in diameter worked using liquid nitrogen. The probe was applied to the tumour for one minute on 3 occasions to the same area. These patients were not considered suitable for surgery and none had received chemotherapy. Four had received radiotherapy for small cell carcinoma and presented with recurrent growths. In one case a cylindroma was engulfing the distal trachea, the carina and main bronchus. A reduction in tumour volume was achieved in five out of the six cases.

The first detailed report also came from the Mayo Clinic and Mayo Foundation [12]. The study group consisted of 28 patients. The most frequent diagnosis for which cryotherapy was given was squamous cell bronchogenic carcinoma. Except in one patient, all conventional forms of surgical and radiation therapy had been attempted, but disease apparently limited to the thorax still persisted. One patient with a cylindroma and one with tracheopathia osteoplastica had cryotherapy as the primary treatment. One patient had recurrent bronchial carcinoid tumour following lobectomy and previous electrocautery treatments. One other patient had previous radiation therapy for carcinoma of oesophagus, but a mediastinal nodal metastasis invaded the trachea and compromised the lumen of the airway.

The 55 cm probe, with interchangeable tips, used liquid nitrogen. The temperature of the tip was reduced to approximately − 160° C and the probe was inserted and applied to the tumour for two minutes. Three freeze-thaw cycles were carried out. Generally, bronchoscopic examination was repeated 4 to 8 weeks later to evaluate the results and also to repeat cryotherapy. The results of this study are summarized in Table 1.

Fifteen of the patients (54 %) obtained benefit from cryotherapy. Two patients with bronchogenic carcinoma have had a long term excellent response (5 years nine months for one and 4 years for the other) and may be cured. Among these patients was the one with cylindroma, who experienced excellent initial shrinkage of tumour and relief of symptoms that was sustained for 2 and a half years. However, in this study there

Table 1. Sanderson — Brochoscopic cryotherapy : results

	Patients	
	N°	%
Favourable result	15	54
Local tumour control	8	
Decreased bleeding	4	
Improved airway patency	3	
No benefit	13	46

was no mention of the efficacy of cryotherapy in the treatment of osteoplastic tracheal lesions.

During cryotherapy, no patient experienced any change in rhythm or any signs of myocardial ischaemia during the procedure. Two patients died, one from a haemoptysis 5 days following cryosurgery for a voluminous friable haemorrhagic tumour of the left main bronchus. It is possible that the cryotherapy was to blame but no autopsy was carried out. The other patient died from acute respiratory failure, presumably due to oedema in the airway, in a patient with previous right pneumonectomy and radiation therapy, who had recurrent squamous cell carcinoma at the stump that extended across the carina and into the proximal left main bronchus. These authors concluded that the ideal indication for cryosurgery is in small superficial tumours of the trachea or main bronchi. Nevertheless, in selected patients with endobronchial tumours in whom the other local therapeutic modalities have been exhausted or in whom further surgical or radiation therapy is not feasible, bronchoscopic cryotherapy does serve as a good alternative for palliation and even long term tumour control.

After an experimental study Rodgers et al [13] published their results of cryotherapy for non-neoplastic stenosis of the large airways. The first report concerned 17 patients [14] and the second concerned 27 patients [15] treated between 1976 to 1981 for stenoses resistant to other forms of treatment : dilatations, alone or in association with sub-mucosal injections of corticosteroids, or stents. The laser was never used however. The patients ages ranged from 3 months to 42 years with a predominance of patients in the younger age group. The cryoprobe (Frigitronics of Connecticut) employed for these procedures was an instrument designed specifically for use through a paediatric endoscope. It measured 43 cm in length and 3 mm in outside diameter, with an angled shaft to allow direct vision during use, and used nitrous oxide as a coolant source. The region of frozen tissue was resected with endoscopic biopsy forceps immediately after thawing of the tissue interface, which allowed removal of cryoprobe. Usually, two or three applications of the cryoprobe were necessary to treat 180 degrees of the tracheal circumference ; following cryoresection, lesions in the subglottic and distal tracheal regions were injected submucosally with triamcinolone acetonide. With very severe strictures in the subglottic region and proximal trachea, endotracheal stenting was employed. All patients underwent endoscopy at four to six week intervals, and further cryotherapy was applied as necessary. When complete relief of airway obstruction had been demonstrated by endoscopy, the patients were extubated. Follow-up endoscopy was repeated at four weeks and three months after extubation to assure continued relief. The obstructions to the airway were divided into three anatomical locations : subglottic stenosis, tracheal strictures and main bronchi strictures. Sixteen lesions treated by cryotherapy were in the subglottic region. Six were thought to be of congenital origin, all in infants symtomatic from birth and requiring tracheostomies for airway management. Each of these infants had cryotherapy instituted in the first year of life when dilatations had failed to relieve the obstruction. The remainder of the subglottic stenoses resulted from endotracheal intubation. The ages of the patients with acquired lesions ranged between 6 months to 30 years. In this entire group there were 4 deaths not related to cryotherapy (3 cardiac malformations and one destruction of a tracheostomy). One patient was lost to follow-up. Of the remaining 11, 6 had been successfully relieved of their airway obstruction and were extubated. The follow-up period after extubation in these patients extends from 1 to 6 years (median, 4 years) and in no case has there been evidence of recurrence of the subglottic narrowing. In 3 other cases, the area of airway narrowing has been completely relieved by cryotherapy but the patients remain intubated. Severe tracheomalacia has prevented successful intubation in 2, and in the third, neurological impairment delayed the extubation. In 2 patients with subglottic strictures, cryotherapy was unsuccessful in relieving the airway obstruction.

Ten patients had treated for tracheal strictures.

The ages of these patients ranged between 1 year and 42 years, and all their lesions were acquired. Four patients were treated for fibrogranulation tissue. In each case the lesion responded to a single application of cryotherapy. Of the remaining 6 patients, 5 had tracheal strictures secondary to endotracheal intubation and in 1 patient the cause of the stricture could not be determined. In these 6 patients an average of 2 applications of cryotherapy was necessary to achieve relief of airway obstruction. In this group, 9 patients were successfully extubated, with follow-up periods ranging between 2 and 6 years following closure of the tracheostomy. In no case was there any endoscopic evidence of recurrence of stricture.

Three patients were treated for strictures of the mainstem bronchus. Cryotherapy was unsuccessful in one of these who had a combination of fibrous stricture and bronchomalacia.

With these results, the authors advocated the efficacy of the technique, the simplicity of the equipment and the relative ease with which it could be used by most doctors who were familiar with endoscopic techniques.

Synthesis

We have deliberately included these early studies because they are fundamental to the subject and are not well known either by cryotherapists in general or chest physicians in particular. They demonstrate the efficacy of cryotherapy in the tracheo-bronchial tree and they also highlight the important advantages vis-à-vis other techniques ; absence of perforation or stenosis, and a restoration of normal respiratory mucosa. Thus cryosurgery has a role to play in bronchial pathology in man. The indications are varied as we have seen in the preceding studies with treatment of benign or malignant tumours and some non tumoral stenoses during which the absence of haemorrhagic complications has been generally underlined. But both these experimental and clinical studies were carried out by only 2 or 3 teams and did not create an impact. The technique was not diffused and indeed it virtually disappeared until rediscovered in Europe but this time with greater success.

There are probably several reasons for this : the studies were carried out on very small numbers ; there was little information available and the technique was not taught to any other users ;

the equipment was probably not very reliable and the manufacturers could not see a potential market for endoscopic cryoprobes. Finally the concomittant arrival of the laser with its media support and undoubted efficacy was a formidable rival to cryotherapy. With hindsight, we think that the treatment of benign stenoses by Rodgers et al. [15] using a cryotherapy-resection with forceps technique, is probably better indicated for a laser rather than cryotherapy or perhaps a combination of the two techniques.

The temperatures achieved by Sanderson [12] of $-160°$ C using a liquid nitrogen cryoprobe and by Rodgers [15] of $-80°$ C using a nitrous oxide cryoprobe are in fact the temperatures achieved in the cryoprobe tip and although they indicate the correct functioning of the cryoprobe the tissues are frozen at considerably less cold temperatures.

Certain fundamental studies must be repeated in order to standardise the method for clinical use depending on the equipment used and the type of liquid coolant. Information needs to be provided on the optimum length of time and number of freeze-thaw cycles applied to a given area in order to obtain the maximal destructive effect on cancerous cells. The speed of freezing and thawing, the temperature differential in the ice-ball and, in relation to the cryoprobe, the relationship between the depth of freezing and various measurements such as thermometry and impedancemetry all need to be established. A correlation between clinical effects and electron microscopy needs to be made and an attempt to codify the method with a view to drawing up a standardized protocol of freeze-thaw times depending on the type of tissue to be treated. Also if one considers the possibility of an immunological effect of freezing there are many studies that could be done in the field of respiratory medicine. Work is being done at present and although the answers are not published in this book at least some questions have been posed and possible avenues of research have been explored.

Finally the indications of cryotherapy must be determined in relation to other methods of relief of bronchial obstruction, namely laser, diathermy and endobrachytherapy, indeed cryotherapy may be used alone or in combination with any of these other techniques. In malignancies the combination of cryotherapy and either chemotherapy or radiotherapy is also worth considering.

Cryotherapy is a cytotoxic procedure and as such should be integrated into the plan of action of treatments for bronchial carcinoma. It should no longer be compared with laser treatment as a simple method of relieving bronchial obstruction but should be considered as a treatment for bronchial neoplasms either alone or in combination with other treatments.

Progress

Around 1984 tracheo-bronchial cryosurgery underwent a renaissance with the coincidental simultaneous publication of several studies in 1986 from three different authors [16-18]. All used cryoprobes driven by nitrous oxide and the conclusions were similar, namely a simple reliable method with no complications. It was used for palliative treatment of bronchial neoplasms and as a curative treatment for certain benign lesions.

In spite of the work by Astesiano [18] in Italy and especially Maiwand [17-20] in England the technique has not been disseminated widely in these two countries. In France, however more and more people are learning the technique, and the information is disseminated by the European Cryosurgery Study Group* and especially the French language respiratory medicine society which has agreed to support a study group within the society [21].

In the face of such demand several practical study courses have been established notably at Chevilly-Larue near Paris where the technique was first perfected in France.

Since 1986 there have been numerous publications on cryotherapy [22-26], papers read at meetings and 5 theses concerning cryotherapy have been published as well as several video films. Patients have also been treated in Belgium, Portugal, Czechoslovakia and Spain [32-34].

At present the cryotherapy equipment is only available in Europe, there are however a large number of American chest physicians who would like to use this equipment and diffuse the technique in their country for the obvious benefit of their patients. Cryotherapy is already used in other disciplines in the United States under the aegis of the American College of Cryosurgery** although at present there is no one in the College who represents respiratory medicine.

---

* European Cryosurgery Study Group, 8, rue Ambroise-Croizat, 03100 Montluçon, France.
** American College of Cryosurgery, 1567 Maple Avenue, PO Box 3116, Evanston, Illinois 60204-3116, USA

References

1. Bradley PF (1986) Cryosurgery of the maxillo-facial region. CRC Press, Boca Raton, Florida
2. Gage AA, Greene GW, Neiders ME, Emmings FG (1969) Freezing bone without excision. An experimental study of bone cell destruction and manner of regrowth in dogs. JAMA 196 : 770
3. Grana L, Kidd J, Swenson O (1969) Cryogenic techniques within tracheobronchial tree. J Cryosurg 2 : 62-67
4. Thomford NR, Wilson WH, Blackburn ED, Pace WG (1970) Morphological changes in canine trachea after freezing. Cryobiology 7 : 19-28
5. Skivolocki WP, Pace WG, Thomford NR (1971) Effect of cryotherapy on tracheal tumours in rats. Arch Surg 103 : 341-343
6. Neel HG, Farrell KH, Payne WS, De Santo LW, Sanderson DR (1973) Cryosurgery of respiratory structures 1. Cryonecrosis of trachea and bronchus. Laryngoscop 83 : 1062-1071
7. Neel HB, Farrell KH, Payne WS, De Santo LW (1974) Cryosurgery of respiratory structures 2. Cryonecrosis of the lung. Laryngoscope 84 : 417-426
8. Gorenstein A, Neel HB, Sanderson DR (1976) Transbronchoscopic cryosurgery of respiratory strictures. Experimental and clinical studies. Ann Otol Rhinol Laryngol : 85-670
9. Carpenter RJ, Neel HB, Sanderson DR (1977) Cryosurgery of bronchopulmonary structures. An approach to lesions inaccessible to the rigid bronchoscope. Chest 72 : 279-284
10. Carpenter RJ, Neel HB, Sanderson DR (1977) Comparison of endoscopic cryosurgery and electrocoagulation of bronchi. Trans Am Acad Ophtalmol Otolaryngol 84 : 313-323
11. Gage AA (1968) Cryotherapy for cancer. In cryosurgery. Rand R, Rinfret A and Von Leden H, Editors 376-387. Thomas Charles C., Publisher Springfield — Illinois
12. Sanderson DR, Neel HB, Payne NS, Woolner LB (1975) Cryotherapy of bronchogenic carcinoma. Report of a case. Mayo Clin Proc : 435-437
13. Sanderson DR, Neel HB, Fontana RS (1981) Bronchoscopic cryotherapy. Ann Otol 90 : 354-358
14. Rodgers BM, Rosenfeld M, Talbert JL (1977) Endobronchial cryotherapy in the treatment of tracheal strictures. J Pediatr Surg 12 : 443-450
15. Rodgers BM, Talbert JL (1978) Clinical application of endotracheal cryotherapy. J Pediatr Surg 13 : 662-666
16. Rodgers BM, Moazam PF, Talbert JL (1983) Endotracheal cryotherapy in the treatment of refractory airway strictures. Ann Thor Surg 35 : 52-57
17. Homasson JP, Renault P, Angebault M, Bonniot JP, Bell NJ (1986) Bronchoscopic cryotherapy for airway strictures caused by tumors. Chest 90 : 159-164
18. Maiwand MO (1986) Cryotherapy for advanced carcinoma of the trachea and bronchi. Br Med J 293 : 181-182
19. Astesiano A, Aversa S, Ciotta D, Galietti F, Gandolfi G, Giorgis GE, Doliaro A, Scappaticci E, Pepino E (1986) Distruzione crioterapica dei tumori invasivi tracheobronchiali. Casistica personale. Min Med 77 : 2159-2162
20. Homasson JP (1989) Cryotherapy in pulmonology today and tomorrow. Eur Resp J 2 : 799-801
21. Walsh DA, Maiwand MO, Nath AR, Lockwood P, Llyod MH, Saab M Bronchoscopic cryotherapy for advanced bronchial carcinoma
22. Blanc-Jouvan F, Eichler B, Homasson JP, Vergnon JM (1989) Recommandations à propos des contre-indications et précautions d'emploi de la cryothérapie bronchique par sonde souple. Rev Mal Resp : 6-479
23. Bonniot JP, Angebault M, Roullier A, Homasson JP (1986) Traitement des granulomes trachéo-bronchiques par cryothérapie. Presse Med : 15-677
24. Angebault M, Bonniot JP, Baud D, Farlet D, Homasson JP (1987) La cryothérapie dans le traitement des obstructions trachéo-bronchiques d'origine tumorale. Rev Pneumol Clin 43 : 13-18
25. Vergnon JM, Boucheron S, Bonamour D, Fournel P, Emonot A (1987) Destruction endobronchique des lésions tumorales : laser ou cryothérapie ? Rev Pneumol Clin 43 : 19-25
26. Eichler B, Savy FP, Melloni B, Germouty J (1988) Désobstruction tumorale trachéo-bronchique par cryothérapie souple. Presse Med 17 : 2138-2139
27. Roden S, Homasson JP (1989) Une nouvelle indication de la cryothérapie endobronchique : l'extraction de corps étrangers. Presse Med 18 : 897
28. Farlet D (1986) Cryothérapie en pneumologie. Thesis. Pierre et Marie Curie University, Paris
29. Savy FP (1988) Cryothérapie bronchique. Effets du traitement endoscopique de 111 lésions bronchiques par cryothérapie à l'aide de sondes souples ou semi-rigides. Thesis. Limoges University
30. Donne E (1988) Cryobiopsies pleurales et pulmonaires lors de thoracoscopie. Thesis. Paris Sud University
31. Guichenez P (1989) Expérience de 3 ans de la cryothérapie endobronchique par sonde semi-rigide. A propos de 107 traitements. Saint-Étienne University
32. Rayel-Boisdron C (1989) La cryothérapie en pathologie trachéo-bronchique. Thesis. Nancy University
33. Pesek M, Bruha PF, Straus J (1988) First experience with endoscopic cryosurgery. Eur Resp J 1 (suppl 2) : 342s
34. Pesek M, Simecek C, Bruha F (1890) Kryokoagulation in der Behandlung von Bronchialtumoren — Z Erkrank. Atm Org 175 : 126-131
35. Luna Sabate D, Sebastian Quetglas F, Romay Diez F, Luque Diez R, Teller Justes P, Mugica Atorrasagasti N (1988) La criocirurgia endoscopica en el tratamiento de las obstrucciones traqueobronquiales. Arch Bronconeumol 24 (suppl 1) : 52-53

Tracheo-bronchial endoscopic cryotherapy

Jean-Paul Homasson

Material

Endoscope equipment

Tracheo-bronchial cryotherapy may be carried out using rigid, semi-rigid or flexible cryoprobes. The rigid and semi-rigid cryoprobes are used with a rigid bronchoscope and the flexible cryoprobes are used in the operative lumen of a fibre optic bronchoscope.

The choice of rigid bronchoscope is not important but the operative lumen must have a diameter large enough for the cryoprobe and the rigid optic system (Fig. 1). This means a minimum diameter of 8 mm for a rigid adult bronchoscope.

The main marques used are Storz (Tuttlingen, Germany), Wolf (Knittligen, Germany) and Efer (Paris, France). The last of these is particularly well adapted for operational endoscopy, not only for cryosurgery but also for laser work and in-serting stents. Wolf have refined a rigid optic system using a bayonet adaptor which has a diameter of 7 mm, it also contains a lumen of 3 mm diameter which is sufficient for the passage of cryoprobes. With all these systems cryosurgery may be carried out under direct vision.

The efficacy of a cryoprobe depends in part on its diameter, thus if it is necessary to use a fibre optic bronchoscope the operative lumen must be as large as possible, around 3mm. At the handle end of the bronchoscope the operative canal should be wide enough to allow a smooth introduction of the cryoprobe without having to force it. This means that the handle of the bronchoscope is suitably angled bearing in mind that the rigid metal tip of the cryoprobe is about 10 mm. Most fibre optic bronchoscopes accept the flexible cryoprobe but the Pentax FB 19 H is particularly well suited and is able to withstand prolonged freezing times. We have never encountered any distortion of the optical equipement by cold, however with other marques of endoscopes

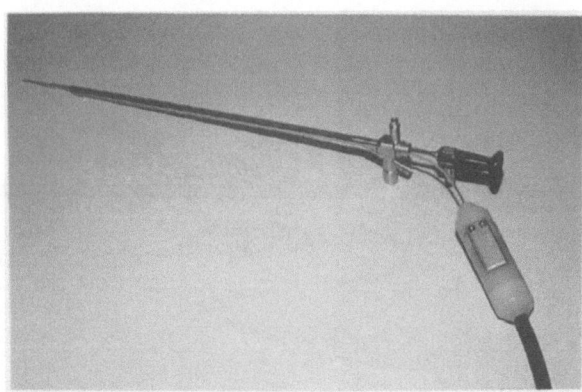

Fig. 1. Semi-rigid cryoprobe (DATE) introduced into a rigid bronchoscope

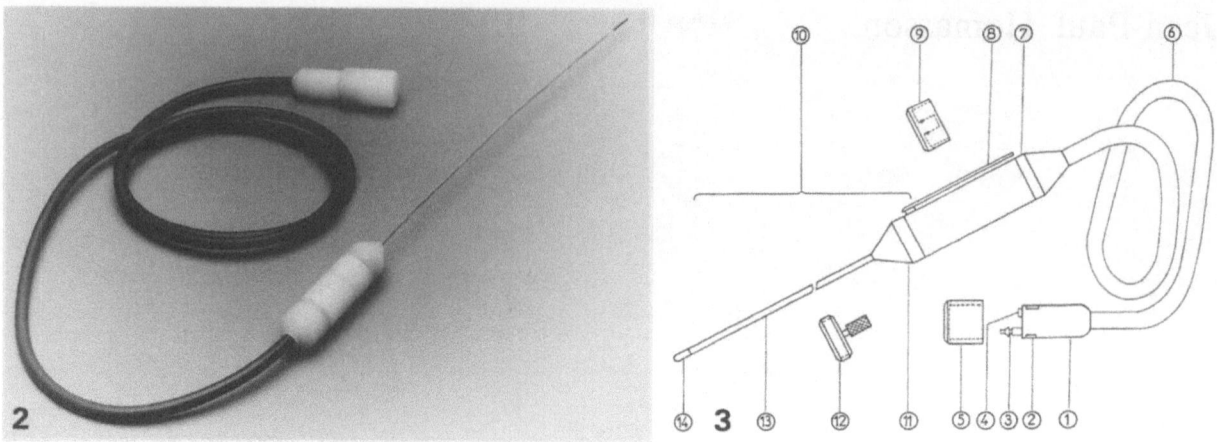

Fig. 2. Semi-rigid cryoprobe (DATE)

Fig. 3. Semi-rigid cryoprobe (LP 400) (DATE). *1* Connecting mechanism, *2* Gas outlet, *3* Pneumatic connector, *4* Coaxial, *5* Connection shield, *6* Tube with liquid gas, *7* Handle, *8* Reheating lever, *9* Sterilising plug (for tube), *10* Removable probe, *11* Threaded hood, *12* Sterilising plug (probe), *13* Semi-rigid shaft, *14* Tip of probe

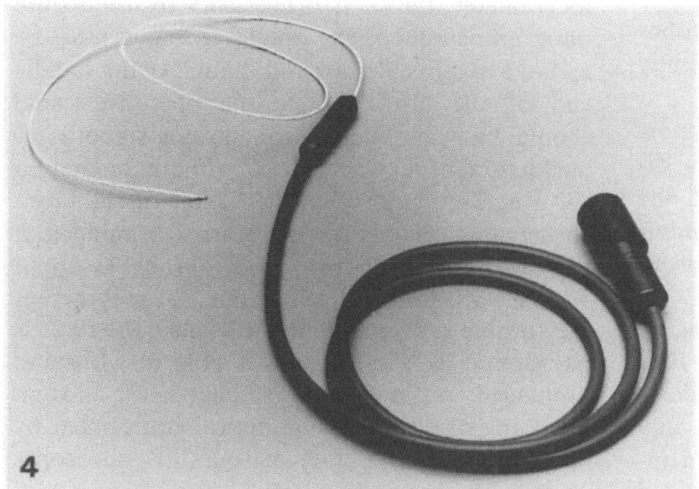

Fig. 4. Flexible cryoprobe (DATE)

Fig. 5. Thermal exchanges before and after release of gas

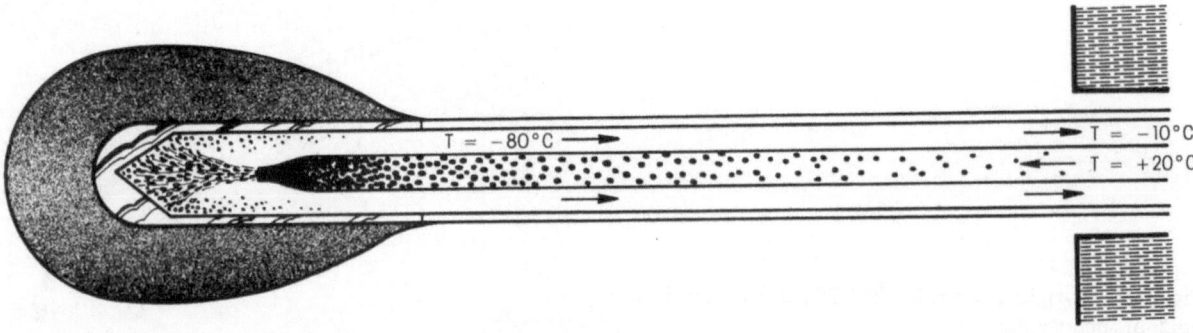

it is worth verifying with the manufacturers that the equipment may be used at low temperatures. The flexible cryoprobe cools the entire endoscope and this effect may be increased with retrofreezing if the cryoprobe is defective or has been used for prolonged freezing cycles.

There are no special accessories needed beyond those normally used for bronchoscopy, namely aspirators, forceps and haemostatic drugs. Photographic recording is essential and a video camera with recording facilities is always desirable.

Endoscopic cryoprobes

At present most cryoprobes employed in tracheo-bronchial cryotherapy use nitrous oxide to cool them according to the Joule-Thomson effect (release of a gas from a high to low pressure zone). The probes have been made small enough to pass down the operative channel of a bronchoscope.

DATE model (La Motte d'Aveillans, France)

Two main cryoprobes have been developed, semi rigid and flexible.

a) *The semi-rigid probe* (Fig. 2) measures 60 cm long and has an external diameter of 3 mm. It has a metal shaft which divides the probe into two lumens for the passage of liquid to the tip of the probe and back. The shaft is covered throughout its entire length by a sheath of Teflon except the last cm which is the metal tip of the probe. It can be bent easily provided the radius of the curvature is greater than 5 cm. It is possible to sterilize the probe in an autoclave up to 130° C or with ethyl ether or by soaking in antiseptic.

The probe may be dismantled from the handle (Fig. 3) and the tube conveying the nitrous oxide may be disconnected at the locating cone in Figure 3. This mechanism allows various probes to be used for different purposes (bronchial cryotherapy or shorter probes for lung or pleural cryobiopsies) or even in different disciplines. The probes may also be sterilized separately from the nitrous oxide tube. The after-sales service is mainly provided for the fragile probe itself.

The supply of nitrous oxide to the probe is regulated by a valve mechanism controlled pneumatically by a pedal. The handle which is in line with the probe has a lever which can cut off the escape of nitrous oxide thus maintaining a high pressure in the probe. When the nitrous oxide comes into contact with the cold wall of the tip of the probe the gas liquifies releasing the latent heat of condensation. The temperature of the tip of the probe rises above − 10° C. This rapid re-heating of the probe enables an almost immediate release of the probe from the frozen tissue.

b) *The flexible cryoprobe* — This is also detachable from the handle. It is 1 300 cm long and the diameter is between 2-3 mm (Fig. 4). The flexible cryoprobe is unable to withstand the same high pressure of nitrous oxide as the rigid probe and a mechanism for regulating the pressure to around 42 bars has been developed. The supply of nitrous oxide is regulated by a similar system as for the rigid probe, again controlled pneumatically by a pedal. The flexible sheath is made of plastic and will not support the high pressure achieved when the gas return is interrupted thus the facility of reheating the tip of the probe to release it from the frozen tissue is not possible. This will inevitably prolong any procedure as one has to wait for natural thawing to occur after each freeze.

In addition the plastic sheath cannot be used in the autoclave although immersion up to a temperature of 50° C is possible.

Table 1 illustrates the thermal performance of some of the flexible probes.

The problem of thermal exchanges between the high pressure fluid coming from the gas bottle and the cold fluid returning via the exhaust was examined to avoid any possible damage to the endoscope by the cold. In normal use the temperature of cold gas returning from the cryoprobe tip is between − 80° C to − 10° C for the first two centimetres of the tube. Droplets at around + 20° C form in the high pressure fluid going towards the exhaust orifice (Fig. 5).

ERBE Equipment (Tübingen, Germany)

This company also make two probes : rigid and flexible.

Table 1. Freezing power of flexible probes (DATE — France)

Diameter mm	3.0	2.6	2.3	2.0
Frozen volume t ≤ 1 min (cm³)	0.60	0.40	0.25	0.18
Thermal power	3.5	2.4	1.5	1.0
Thermal flux	3.2	2.6	2.5	2.1

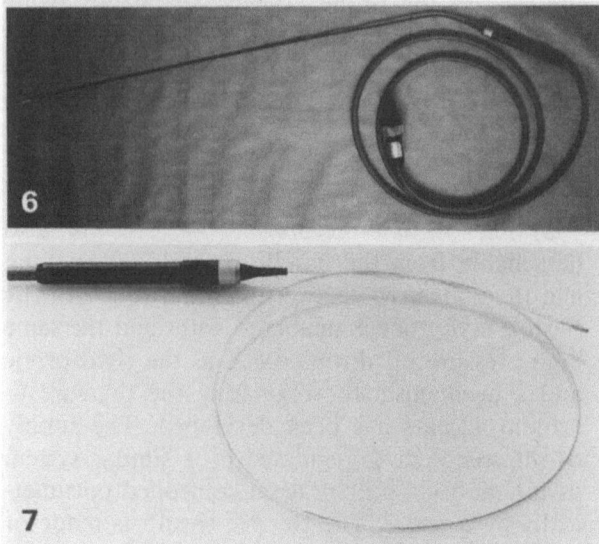

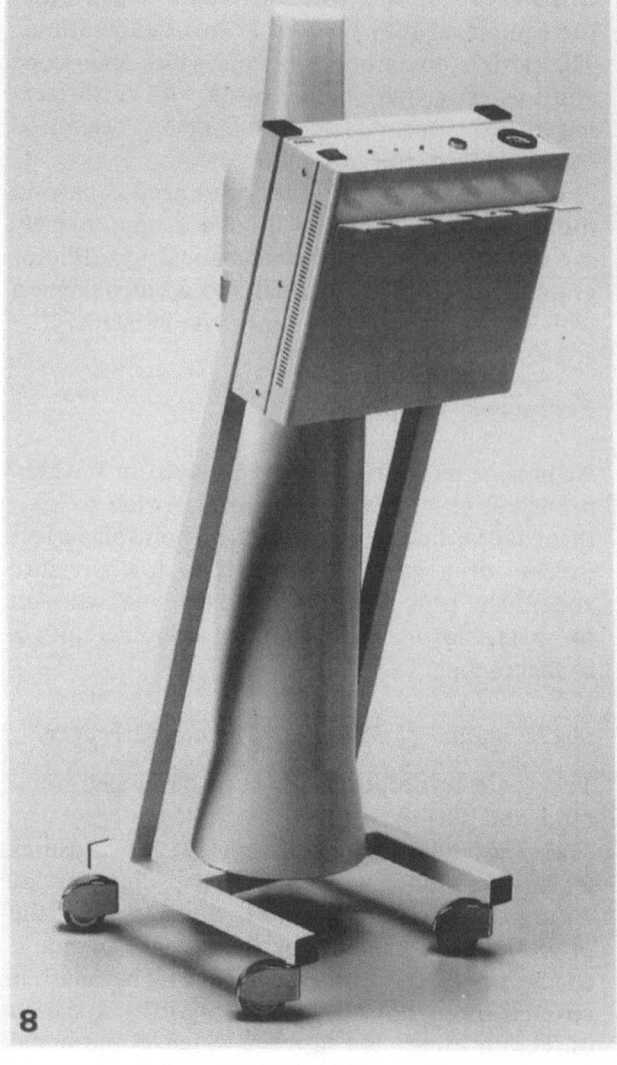

Fig. 6. Rigid cryoprobe (ERBE)

Fig. 7. Flexible cryoprobe (ERBE)

Fig. 8. ERBE cryo unit (Erbocryo CA)

The rigid probe is 52 cm long with an external diameter of 2,5 mm (Fig. 6). It is isolated along its entire length except for the metal tip which is 10 mm long. It is operated by a pedal system and the tip becomes free immediately the pedal is released by cutting the flow of gas. The probe, however is not detachable from the gas delivery tube. Sterilization is carried out by soaking in a solution of glutaraldehyde or by other methods such as ethylene chloride, formalin, etc.

The flexible probe measures 80 cm and may have an external diameter of either 2.2 mm, 2.7 mm or 2.9 mm depending on the diameter of the operative channel of the endoscope being used. The metal tip is 7 mm long (Fig. 7).

Both the rigid and flexible probes form an integral part of the endoscopic cryosurgery equipment Erbocryo CA (Fig. 8).

Spembly equipment (Andover, England)

At present Spembly make a rigid probe which measures 45 cms and has an external diameter of 4 mm (Fig. 9). Two versions are available : with or without an integral thermocouple (copper-constantan) incorporated in the tip of the probe.

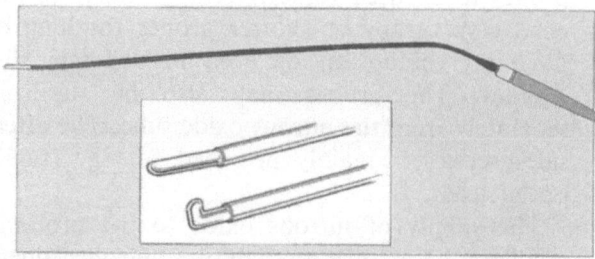

Fig. 9. Spembly medical cryoprobes : bronchial small angle probe 40-27 H7L, bronchial, right angle probe 40-FAB 10 L

The measurement of the temperature at the tip of the probe is a good indication that the probe is working properly. These probes have the advantage of being able to function using different types of gas : CO_2 which is cheap though not as efficient as nitrous oxide ; nitrous oxide « medical quality » which is approximately double the price of CO_2 and purified nitrous oxide which is even more expensive. These probes may be sterilised either in an autoclave or else by soaking. Spembly is considering developing a flexible cryoprobe.

Chirana Company Brno

This Czechoslovakian probe measures 4 mm in diameter with a tip of 5 mm diameter and is 50 cms long. It has a cooling capacity of 30 W. The probe is angled at 25° C to allow direct vision when it is inserted into the bronchoscope.

Cryogens

It comes in a bottle in the liquid state and the pressure depends on the temperature of the bottle and obviously the ambient temperature where it is stored (see Table 2 in chapter on Cryogens). However if the bottle is stored outside in winter it is sometimes necessary to allow it to warm up before it has a sufficient pressure for use. Likewise it should not be stored close to a source of heat.

The bottle must be in the upright position when in use in order to draw from the gaseous fraction. It is fitted with a manual regulator which ensures a steady supply of pressurized gas at about 40-50 bars. When the nitrous oxide is released it cools to a temperature of around − 80° C and is in a partially liquid state. It forms a mist of fine droplets which impinge on the inner surface of the metal tip of the probe and cool it to around − 60° C. When the probe is immersed in saline or forced into tissue an ice ball forms around the tip (Fig. 10). The temperature in this ball depends on the distance from the probe, the temperature rising towards the periphery of the ice ball.

After 20 seconds of freezing in a saline solution at 37° C the temperature 1 mm from the probe is around − 20° C whilst the ice in contact with the probe will be of the order of − 40° C. The droplets which come into contact with the metal tip of the probe are vaporized and the gas passes by the return tube of the probe and escapes at the exhaust vent in the handle.

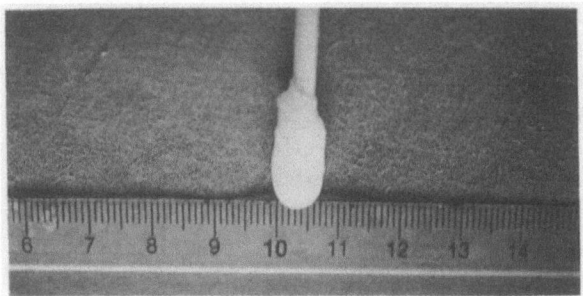

Fig. 10. Cryoprobe with ice ball

Table 2. Cryoprobes

Make	Country of manufacture	Type	Length (cm)	Diameter (mm)	Length tip of probe (mm)	Coolant source	Controls*			Sterilisation		
							P	Z	T	Autoclave	Gas	Soaking
DATE	France	Semi rigid	60	3.0	10	N2 0 Cryo	×	×		×	×	×
		Flexible	1 300	2.0-2.3 2.6-3.0	10	N₂0 Cryo	×	×			×	×
ERBE	Germany	Rigid	52	2.5	10	N₂0 Cryo	×			×	×	×
		Flexible	80	2.2-2.4 2.7-	7	N₂0 Cryo	×				×	×
Spembly	UK	Rigid	45	2.0-3.0	10	N₂0 Cryo N₂0 CO₂	×		×	×	×	×
Chirana	Czecho-slovakia	Rigid	50	4	5	Liquid N₂						

* P : control of pressure at bottle, Z : impedance, T : temperature at tip of probe

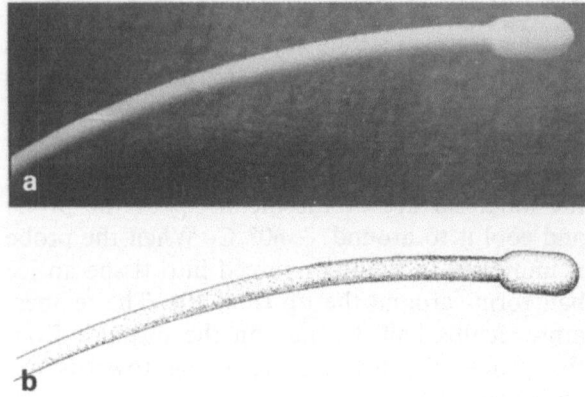

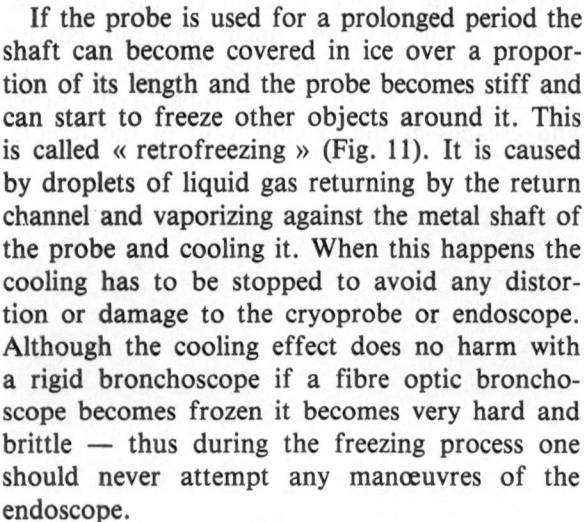

Fig. 11 a, b. Retrofreezing

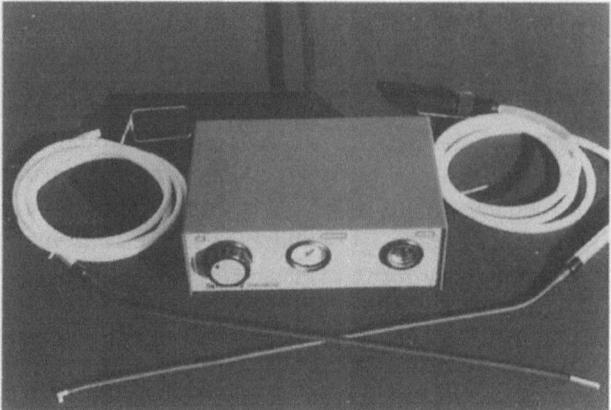

Fig. 12. Spembly medical cryoconsole with cryoprobes

If the probe is used for a prolonged period the shaft can become covered in ice over a proportion of its length and the probe becomes stiff and can start to freeze other objects around it. This is called « retrofreezing » (Fig. 11). It is caused by droplets of liquid gas returning by the return channel and vaporizing against the metal shaft of the probe and cooling it. When this happens the cooling has to be stopped to avoid any distortion or damage to the cryoprobe or endoscope. Although the cooling effect does no harm with a rigid bronchoscope if a fibre optic bronchoscope becomes frozen it becomes very hard and brittle — thus during the freezing process one should never attempt any manœuvres of the endoscope.

Nitrous oxide produces an almost instant cooling effect and we know that the lower the temperature is below zero and the rapidity with which it achieves this temperature the greater the cryodestructive effect will be.

Monitoring techniques

The endoscope limits the methods of control of freezing and there appears to be no ideal solution. The different methods were discussed in the previous chapter but most of them are not applicable to endoscopic cryotherapy. To be efficacious cryotherapy should destroy all the target tissue and leave the neighbouring tissue intact, however there are two factors which need to be considered. Firstly the volume of tissue destroyed does not correspond exactly to the area which is frozen and secondly it is impossible to gauge accurately the depth of freezing within a ball of frozen tissue.

The empirical method relies on the experience of the operator and with some cryoprobes it is the only way of monitoring the freezing process. He relies on the change in colour and consistency of the frozen tissue and the length of freezing is also based on his experience. Using rigid or semi-rigid probes this is usually around 30 seconds for each freeze-thaw cycle. The thaw phase is almost immediate when probes with a system of reheating are used, but with the flexible probes, although the freezing time is comparable the spontaneous thawing is almost as long as the freezing time, thus the whole process takes twice as long.

A thermic method of freeze monitoring with implantation of thermocouples in the tumour at the periphery is not practicable with an endoscope. However a thermocouple incorporated in the tip of the cryoprobe as in the Spembly model (Fig. 12) will at least confirm the correct functioning of the cryoprobe. But even this will not give an accurate indication of the temperature achieved in the frozen tissue and the operator will have to rely on his own experience to estimate the length of time of freezing.

At present the only method of monitoring freezing using an endoscope is the bioelectric method proposed by Le Pivert [1-3] and described in a previous chapter, but even this is far from ideal (Fig. 13). It is based on the fact that complete extracellular crystallisation is essential to produce tissue necrosis — this change in physical state of the extracellular milieu during freezing (crystallisation) leads to a change in the impedance of the tissue. When endoscopic cryotherapy is employed the cryoprobe represents one electrode and the other is a metal plate placed in contact with another part of the patient's body. The ice ball which is formed breaks the current between the two electrodes and when a resistance of between 200-500 kΩ is reached this indicates that the cryoprobe is working correctly. Previous studies have been used to correlate the plateau of impedance with the eutectic freezing of tissue.

However, in the experience of chest physicians there appears to be a wide variation in the relation between the levels of the impedance plateau, the length of time of freezing and the extent of the cryodestruction.

Further studies need to be carried out to verify the situation. A repeated number (usually 3) of freeze-thaw cycles in the same site will raise the impedance (Fig. 14) but again the correlation between that and an increased lethal effect occurring further from the cryoprobe has yet to be determined.

Conclusions

Endoscopes are in fact well adapted for cryotherapy and only a few modifications would be desired by some people. The miniaturisation of the cryoprobes and the use of nitrous oxide represent real progress. However it would be nice to see a few more improvements especially in the ergonomics of the equipment, its robustness and methods of monitoring. The flexible cryoprobes are the most delicate and usually less efficient than the rigid or semi-rigid probes. Thus wherever possible we advise the use of a rigid bronchoscope with rigid or semi-stiff probes as to freeze an equivalent volume of tumour with a flexible probe without a reheat facility will take twice as long.

However rigid bronchoscopes are used less often these days as they usually require a general anaesthetic and considerable expertise on the part of the operator.

All the equipment used for cryotherapy is portable and does not take up much space.

The characteristics of the various probes are summarised in Table 2.

Method

Preparation of the patient

Cryotherapy is most often indicated as palliative treatment of a confirmed bronchial carcinoma.

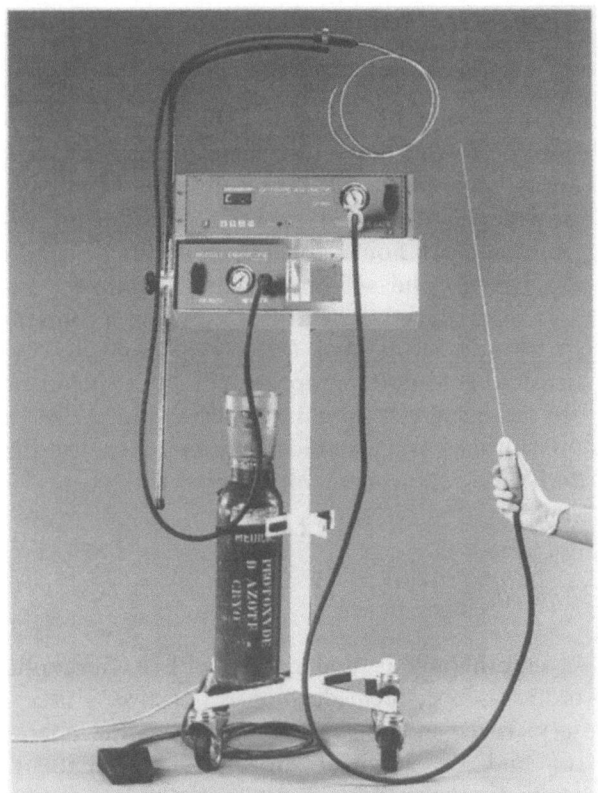

Fig. 13. DATE cryounit with impedance meter

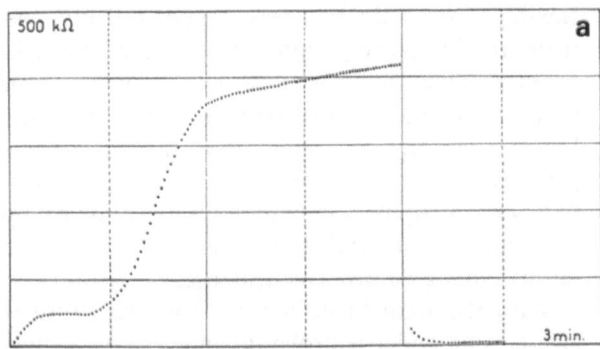

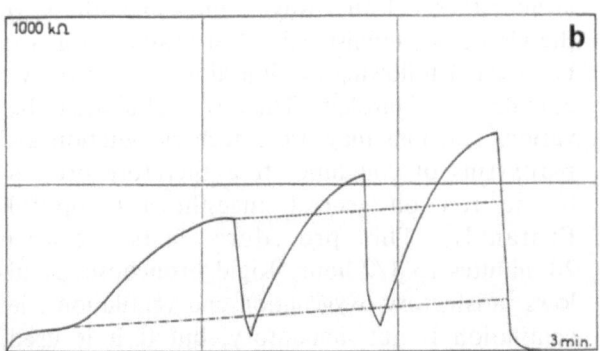

Fig. 14. a Crescent shaped curve of the impedance in relation to time of application of cold in normal saline at ambient temperatures, **b** curve of variation of the impedance during 3 cycles of freezing (normal saline at ambient temperatures)

An initial endoscopy will already have been carried out together with other routine examinations : e.g. radiography, CT scan, full blood count, coagulation studies, blood gasses and respiratory function. This last examination is not always possible in weak and dyspnoeic patients. Anticoagulant therapy is stopped before the examination : 8 hours for low-molecular heparin derivatives and 48 hours for vitamin K antagonists. Reactive oedema following cryotherapy is not severe and the prescription of corticosteroids is not appropriate but any corticotherapy in progress should not be stopped. As a precaution corticosteroids may be given for the 24 hours following cryotherapy of tracheal lesions.

Anaesthesia

If cryotherapy is undertaken with a fibreoptic bronchoscope, premedication is not always necessary. It depends on the preference of the operator and the level of anxiety of the patient. However, when using a fibreoptic bronchoscope with flexible probes the examination often takes a long time : 45 min to 1 h (this is because the flexible probes do not reheat very quickly and their freezing power is inferior to that of the rigid probes. Thus for the destruction of a given volume of tumour the flexible probe wil take longer than the rigid one). For this reason we prefer to administer a premedication with diazepam and atropine sulphate. This is followed by local anaesthesia with lignocaine at 5 % for the larynx and 2 % for tracheal use.

With the rigid bronchoscope the procedure is carried out under neuroleptic analgesia or general anaesthesia. Either way, a local anaesthesia of the glottis is administered. Most examinations can be effected following i.v. injections of one or two ampules of midazolam. There is total amnesia but various reactions may occur such as agitation and paroxysms of coughing. It is therefore preferable to rely on general anaesthesia (Propofol-Fentanyl). The procedure lasts between 20 minutes to 1/2 hour. Rigid bronchoscopy allows satisfactory oxygenation and ventilation : jet ventilation is not mandatory, but if it is used, ventilation is with a frequency of 120/min, with an inspiratory ratio to total time (I/R) of 30 %, using FIO_2 at 50 %. When combined therapy with laser and cryotherapy is used, the jet is disconnected during the laser treatment as there

would be a serious risk of fire, but the cannula may be used to aspirate smoke. All patients are monitored with an electrocardiogram, and normal saline infusion is used during the procedure. The respiratory function of patients is often precarious, in these cases and it is wise to monitor cutaneous O_2 saturation.

Endoscopy

The fibreoptic endoscope is introduced by the nasal or buccal route with the patient in a semi-seated position with the operator facing him, or alternatively in the supine position, which is often preferable when the procedure is likely to last a long time.

Patients are always in the supine position when a rigid bronchoscope is used because of the general anaesthetic (Fig. 15). In patients with a tracheostomy, the endoscope may be inserted via the tracheostomy.

The operator assesses the lesions to be treated, whether they are haemorrhagic or not ; projecting and/or infiltrating, their position and the extent of stenosis or extrinsic compression that may exist.

If the initial diagnostic endoscopy, was carried out by another operator, they may have made

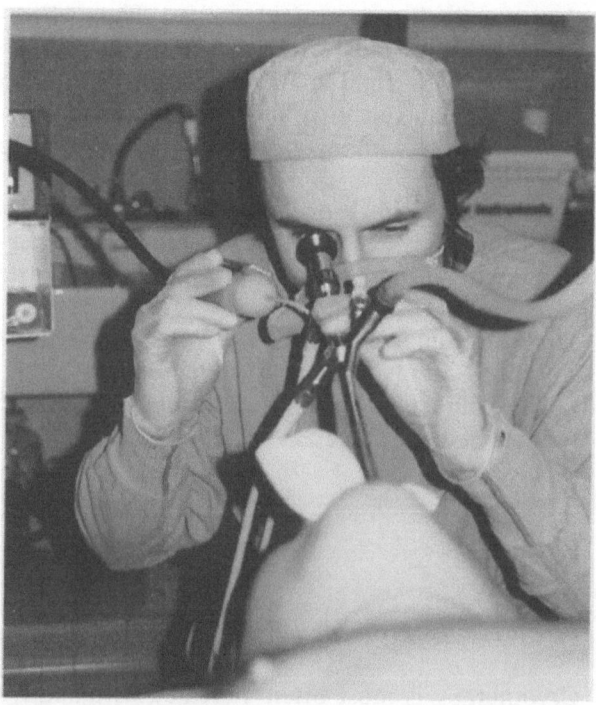

Fig. 15. Cryotherapy using a rigid bronchoscope

different recommendations for the choice of endoscope and probes, and some biopsies may have already been taken. If there is a risk of bleeding, it is preferable to carry out an initial freeze-thaw cycle and biopsy immediately afterwards. In this way the haemostatic properties of cold are utilised, and as will be seen, the quality of specimens obtained for microscopic examination are perfectly satisfactory.

Cryotherapy

The freeze-thaw procedures are carried out under direct vision via the endoscope. The use of flexible probes and a fibreoptic endoscope necessitates certain precautions [1-3]. Due to their fragile nature the flexible probes may not be bent and they should be held as close as possible to the endoscope when passing them through the operative channel. Freezing may only be effected when the portion of the probe emerging from the endoscope is twice as long as the freezing portion (freezing portion included). During the freezing period the fibreoptic endoscope should not be moved and no manœuvres with the tip of the endoscope should be attempted. If the endoscope has to be moved, repositioning may only occur

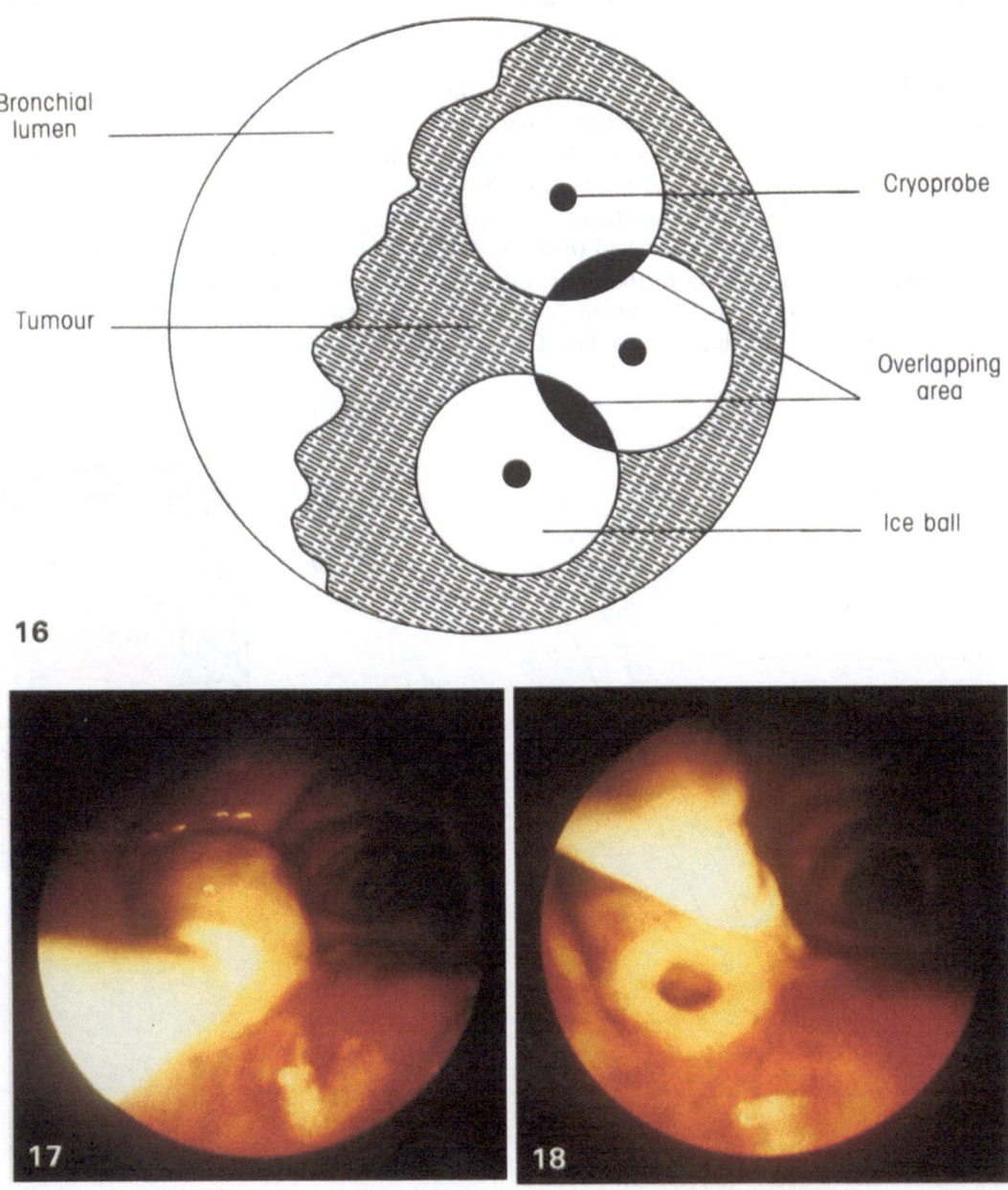

Figs. 16-18. Freezing technique showing overlapping areas

after defrosting. The procedure should be stopped if retrofreezing occurs. The probe must not be removed until complete defrosting has occurred (if not there is a risk of tearing the tissue and causing bleeding).

The method of freezing is the same for flexible, rigid or malleable probes but treatment may vary depending on the appearance of the lesion to be treated.

The most suitable type of lesion is a polypoid one, benign or malignant. The metallic tip of the cryoprobe is pushed into the tumour which produces circumferential freezing of maximal volume. Three freeze-thaw cycles are carried out at each site. The probe is then moved 5-6 mm and another 3 cycles carried out in the adjoining area.. The points of impact are staggered with an overlap of the frozen zone with respect to the previous site. The procedure is continued until the entire visible part of the tumour has been frozen (Figs. 16, 17, 18). If the probe is equipped with a device for measuring the impedance, reheating is effected when a plateau is reached (between 250 and 500 K Ohms, according to the tissue and position of the cryoprobe). Subsequent cycles are commenced when the impedance has fallen to

50 K Ohms but before the probe has become unstuck. With the other probes, the freezing time is around 30 sec per cycle. There is no value in prolonging the freezing beyond this time and indeed research has demonstrated a greater cryodestructive effect using several freeze-thaw cycles rather than a single long freeze.

With infiltrating lesions, cryotherapy can be used with lateral tangential contact (Figs. 19, 20).

It is possible to treat circumferential lesions such as constrictive bronchial stenoses, by placing the cryoprobe at the centre of the stenosis.

Eight to ten days after the first session, a repeat endoscopy is usually performed. This second examination enables assessment of the extent of cryodestruction, removal of any slough and repeat cryotherapy if required. This is generally the case with voluminous tumours. The slough may be removed with forceps, by aspiration, or with the cryoprobe by using the phenomenon of cryo adherence. When this technique is used care must be taken not to damage viable tissue because of the risk of bleeding. If resistance is felt then the probe should not be pulled.

Cryosurgical treatment may require several ses-

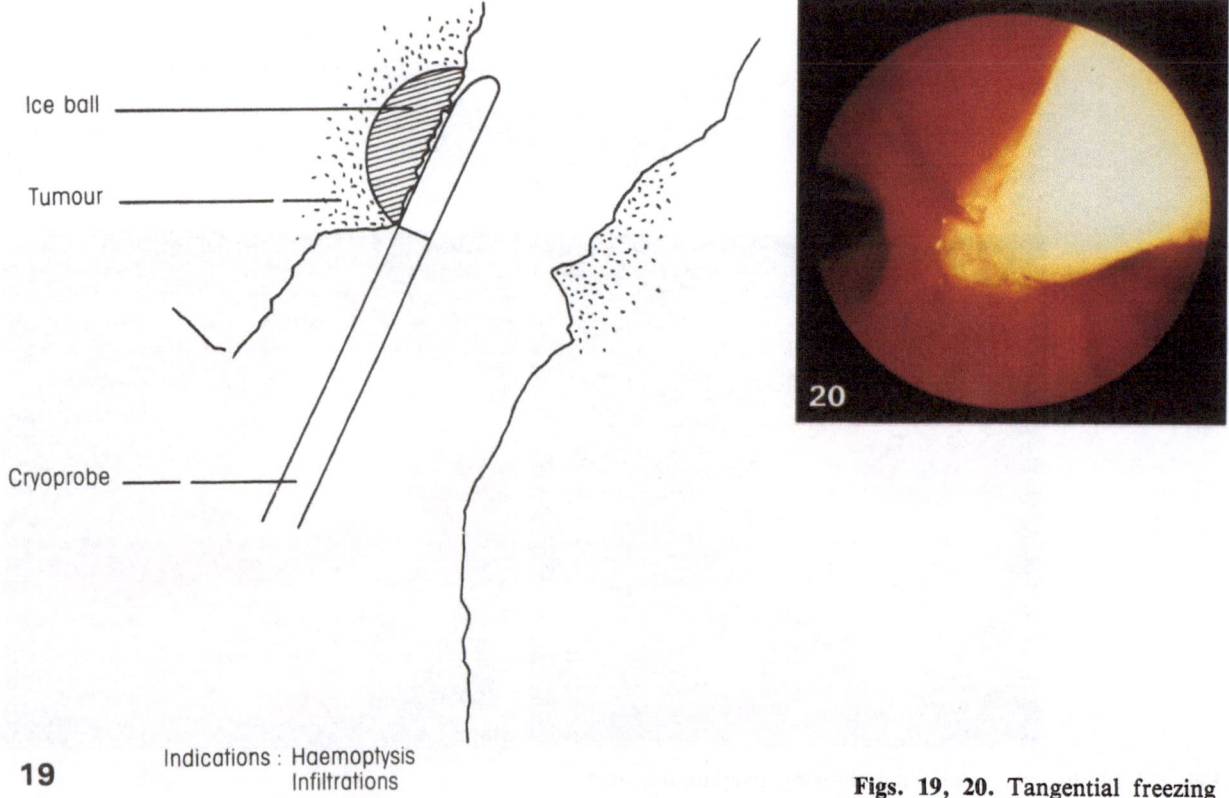

Ice ball

Tumour

Cryoprobe

19   Indications : Haemoptysis
                        Infiltrations

Figs. 19, 20. Tangential freezing

sions. Each session is repeated at 8-15 days intervals according to the results obtained. Several tumours may be treated at the same session.

Post-operative care

Cryotherapy as such does not require any particular immediate follow-up care. If the treatment is carried out using a fibreoptic endoscope, with or without premedication, the patient can return home the same day. In certain cases after a general anaesthetic it is prudent to keep the patient under medical surveillance for 24 hours.

In patients with respiratory insufficiency, blood gases will indicate the need for supplementing O_2 therapy.

Experience has shown that radiography immediately after therapy is not essential. However, occasionally rapid relief of a bronchial obstruction may be achieved by perforation and retraction of tumour tissue after freezing, and reventilation of an area (lobe or lung) may be confirmed with early radiography. This is however a fairly rare occurrence.

Administration of corticosteroids is not routine and is only indicated following treatment of laryngeal or tracheal lesions, where there is a risk of an oedematous reaction.

The haemostatic effect of freezing is often sufficient to stop haemoptysis, but it may be delayed and only occur the day after cryotherapy. Moreover, the trauma caused by the penetrating probe into an already haemorrhagic lesion may temporarily aggravate the bleeding. Haemostatic drugs should then be prescribed. It is prudent to keep the patient under medical observation for 24 hours. But in the large majority of cases haemoptysis immediately following therapy is of no great importance and does not require any treatment.

Conclusion

For a specialist familiar with the use of endoscopy, cryotherapy will not present any particular problems. One of the main advantages is that it is simple and relatively harmless and thus the technique can be mastered easily. At worst, cryotherapy will be ineffective, but the technique is not dangerous and accidental freezing of healthy areas is without consequence. It is enough to quickly reposition the probe to a better position. However, less experienced lung specialists will have to use a rigid bronchoscope.

In our opinion, the fibreoptic endoscope and flexible probes should only be used when it is not possible to use a rigid bronchoscope ; either due to the condition of the patient, or because the position of the lesion renders it inaccessible to a rigid bronchoscope. With current equipment and modern anaesthetic techniques, the rigid bronchoscope should be employed whenever possible rendering the cryotherapy more effective, the duration of the procedure shorter and the safety conditions better (improved ventilation and aspiration).

References

1. Le Pivert P (1974) Cryochirurgie en cancérologie : contribution expérimentale à l'étude de la cryodestruction des cellules tumorales *in vivo*. Thesis Lyon University
2. Le Pivert P, Binder P, Ougier T (1977) Measurement of intratissue bioelectrical low frequency impedance : a new method to predict per-operatively the destructive effect of cryosurgery. Cryobiology 14 : 245-250
3. Le Pivert P (1980) Basic considerations of the cryolesion. In : Ablin RJ (Ed.) Handbook of cryosurgery. Marcel Dekker Inc, New York Basel, pp 15-67

Tracheo-bronchial cryotherapy — Indications and results

Jean-Paul Homasson and Nicholas J. Bell

Indications

The fact that cryotherapy is cheap and easy to use should not alter the indications for its use. For example the relief of an obstruction of a lobar or segmental bronchus will not bring functional improvement, however it may be justified for treating a troublesome symptom such as cough, haemoptysis, infection or perhaps to reduce a field of irradiation if secondary irradiation is envisaged with removal of atelectasis. Quite severe ventilatory obstruction can be well tolerated without any obvious signs of functional deficit and the endobronchial obstruction should not necessarily be removed at all costs. However if a combined treatment of chemotherapy or radiotherapy with cryotherapy were to produce a synergistic response should it not be treated ?

The presenting symptoms or the decision to treat are more important when deciding on cryotherapy rather than the simple endoscopic or radiographic appearance of a lesion. Cryotherapy is not a panacea and it is not only an alternative when other methods have failed, especially laser therapy. It may be considered as a first intention treatment if it is included in the therapeutic protocols of physicians.

Symptom control indications

Cryotherapy may be used to treat symptoms of both malignant and benign lesions. The major symptom amenable to cryotherapy is without doubt haemoptysis caused by a visible lesion. Freezing has a haemostatic effect by causing vasoconstriction and a rapid slowing of the circulation, however this effect is not always immediate and may only occur on the day following cryotherapy. Indeed the penetration of a cryoprobe into a tumour may sometimes be responsible for a transient haemoptysis.

Dyspnoea is also a frequent symptom and patients with bronchial obstructions often have a reduced respiratory reserve and the obstruction of a bronchus may often rapidly aggravate the situation. However at present it must be stated that the fact that cryotherapy has a delayed effect in relieving bronchial obstructions means that it should not be used as emergency treatment in acute respiratory distress, especially if it is due to tracheal obstruction — this clearly remains the domain of laser therapy.

Cough may sometimes be extremely troublesome especially if it occurs at night and prevents sleep.

Stridor is often very disturbing for both the patient and his family as the loud harsh wheeze may easily be heard by anyone in close contact with the patient.

Pain is a common symptom and although there are many causes for it the pain of sudden lobar collapse after total obstruction of a bronchus by tumour may be considerable — this may be relieved by removing the obstruction and allowing reinflation of the affected lobe.

Walsh [1] carried out a prospective study of 33 patients treated with cryotherapy. Each symptom was graded and patients were questioned before and after cryotherapy. All the symptoms except pain were studied and radiography, respiratory function and endoscopy were carried out before and after cryotherapy. Pesek has also completed a study where respiratory function was measured in 23 patients treated with cryotherapy [2].

Indications according to the nature of the lesion

Malignant tumours

Most lesions treated with cryotherapy are malignant tumours either primary bronchial carcinomas or secondary deposits (Fig. 1). Bronchial metastases from renal carcinomas are often very haemorrhagic and the haemostatic effect of cryosurgery is at least as helpful as the relief of obstruction. Small cell carcinoma is rarely amenable to treatment with cryotherapy as it more often causes infiltration and extrinsic compression of a bronchus. The main indications for cryotherapy are polypoid squamous cell or adenocarcinomas — they are also the most frequently encountered carcinomas with a relatively slow progression, representing around 80 % of all indications for cryotherapy. They may be treated several times at weekly or monthly intervals and cryotherapy is clearly indicated for palliation in these cases.

Pre-malignant tumours and tumours of intermediate malignancy

These tumours are much rarer but cryotherapy is often indicated for their treatment, although it is only recognized as an indication when con-

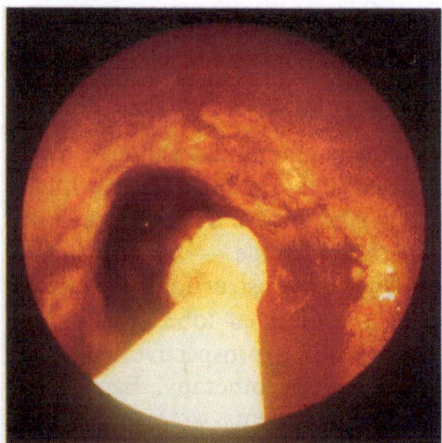

Fig. 1. A malignant tumour of the left main bronchus being treated with cryotherapy

ventional surgery is contra-indicated. If the tumour looks like a carcinoid it is usually frozen first and then a biopsy taken. The haemostatic effect of freezing makes this possible even though these tumours are often haemorrhagic.

Cylindromas are amenable to cryotherapy especially when surgery is contra-indicated as good results may be obtained. Muco-squamous, papillomatous and other tumours of low malignancy may be treated successfully over several sessions especially when surgery is not possible.

Benign tumours

Granulation tissue is an excellent indication for cryotherapy as they are highly cellular and therefore sensitive to the destructive effect of cryotherapy. They are often voluminous and polypoid and may even impede the introduction of tracheostomy cannulae. They are mainly seen in the trachea and can surround a tracheostomy opening or may be present in a bronchial stump following pneumonectomy or lobectomy — they often occur in the presence of suture material, although they are also encountered more rarely with fistulae caused by adenopathies.

Myomas, leiomyomas and Abrikosov tumours sometimes have multiple localizations and may often be the cause of recurrent infections by complete obstruction of a bronchus. In our experience they are a good indication for cryotherapy as they are often situated in distal small bronchi which are inaccessible to laser therapy. They usually require 2 to 3 sessions of cryotherapy for their destruction.

Rodgers [3] was the first person to use cryotherapy in the treatment of non tumour stenosis of the subglottis, trachea or bronchus. These lesions are either congenital or acquired but are usually found in children. The cryotherapy was used in conjuction with forceps dissection but we feel that most of those cases would nowadays be treated with laser or combination of cryotherapy and laser therapy. In reality fibrotic stenoses are not good indications for cryotherapy even if good results have been reported in the past. We have however treated the occasional punctiform stenosis which is often a sequel of tuberculosis — this will often be suppuritive and give rise to breathing difficulties. If the cryoprobe is inserted into the orifice of the cavity and a circumferential freezing obtained this may enlarge the orifice of the cavity permanently and improve drainage of secretions.

Generally speaking, however, fibrous tissue is resistant to the effects of cryotherapy.

Certain benign tumours such as lipomata and chondro-osteoplastica tacheopathia are not amenable to treatment as fat, bone and cartilage are fairly resistant to freezing.

Foreign bodies

Foreign bodies have been extracted in a few cases with success using cryotherapy [4]. This relies on removing friable matter such as inhaled pills or peanuts which would otherwise disintegrate when grasped with forceps and be disseminated into other areas especially as a result of violent movement caused by coughing. When the cryoprobe touches the foreign body it is totally frozen and may be extracted in its entirety (Fig. 2).

The shrinking effect of cold may be used to facilitate the release of a foreign body embedded in an inflammatory bronchial mucosa. This method is possible using a rigid bronchoscope or a fibreoptic one. Some foreign bodies absorb bronchial secretions and are therefore freezable but sometimes this causes technical difficulties as it is not easy to avoid freezing the bronchial wall as well as the foreign body.

This technique may be used to remove blood clots and for extracting slough caused by previous cryotherapy which behave like a foreign body and may be removed in the same way (Fig. 3). However caution must be exercised when pulling a slough in order to avoid tearing viable tissue and thus causing haemorrhage.

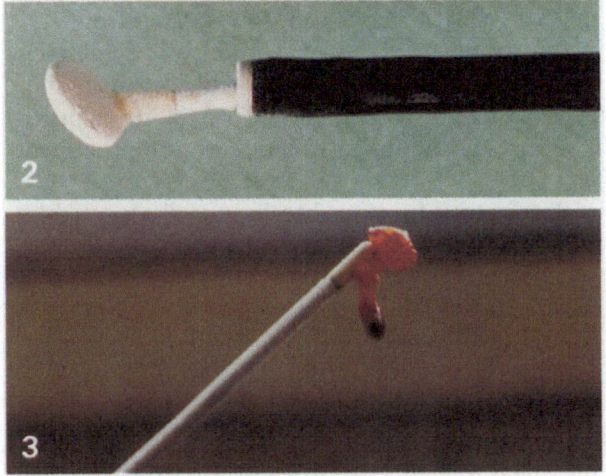

Fig. 2. Retrieval of foreign body (tablet)

Fig. 3. Removal of slough using cryoadherence

Indications according to the site

Where possible all lesions should be treated with a rigid cryoprobe using a rigid bronchoscope, this includes lesions situated in the trachea, main bronchi and the inferior lobar bronchi. Smaller lesions in distal bronchi especially in the upper lobes should be treated using a flexible cryoprobe and a fibre optic bronchoscope. For the same sized tumour, treatment with a rigid probe is much quicker and it is for this reason that we recommend the use of a rigid bronchoscope whenever possible although sometimes it will be necessary to use both, especially when a large obstruction has been cleared to reveal further deposits distally which are inaccessible to the rigid cryoprobe.

Indications according to the type of lesion

If the obstruction is due to tumour, cryotherapy is only indicated if the tumour arises within the bronchi and the soft, polypoid highly cellular lesions which may be easily pierced with the tip of a cryoprobe represent the best indications.

External compression of the bronchi, distortions of the wall of the bronchus and severe tracheal stenoses where the lumen of the trachea is reduced by 50 % or more are not indications for cryotherapy.

Very often cryotherapy will be effective in infiltrative stenoses but for these the cryoprobe is applied tangentially.

Fibrotic or post irradiation stenoses do not respond to cryotherapy but it may be tried without risk as occasional responses do occur.

Micro-invasive carcinoma and carcinoma *in situ* represent interesting indications for cryotherapy which may even be curative but the numbers are so small that it is impossible to draw any firm conclusions even though early results are encouraging. These tumours are discussed in another chapter and form part of a multicentre French trial [5].

There is no obvious difference in sensitivity to cryotherapy between different tumour types but it would seem that small cell carcinomas are a little more sensitive compared to adenocarcinomas but this needs to be confirmed. Melanocytic tumours are particularly sensitive to cryotherapy as treated by dermatologists and veterinary surgeons in animals. However these tumours are extremely rare in the lung and none have been treated with cryotherapy to date.

Results

The results of cryotherapy are judged by several different means, endoscopic appearances, clinical criteria, radiological changes, changes in respiratory function and histological appearances. Most users have generally had good results from using cryotherapy and it is surprising that this method of treatment is not more widely practised in other countries. One of the reasons must be the relatively few papers published — a lot of what has been done is incomplete.

Symptomatic and functional results

All people who have tried this method have obtained a significant improvement or even disappearance of clinical signs of disease after cryotherapy, however only D.A. Walsh and M.O. Maiwand and colleagues [1] have published a precise evaluation. They studied the effects of cryotherapy on dyspnoea, haemoptysis, cough and stridor. Dyspnoea was graded from 0 to 3 according to a modification of the Medical Research Council dyspnea index [6]. 0 — ability to hurry up a hill or upstairs ; 1 — inability to hurry, but able to maintain a normal walking pace on the level for more than six minutes ; 2 — inability to maintain a normal walking pace on the level for more than six minutes without stopping ; 3 — shortness of breath at rest or on minimal exertion such as dressing or undressing. Haemoptysis was graded from 0 to 4 : 0 — no haemoptysis ; 1 — streaks of blood in sputum ; 2 — clots of blood on 4 days or less during the preceding two weeks ; 3 — clots on 5 or more days ; 4 — haemoptysis requiring blood transfusion. Cough was graded from 0 — 2 : 0 — no cough ; 1 — cough not disturbing sleep ; 2 — cough disturbing sleep. Stridor, recorded as present or absent, was defined as inspiratory wheeze associated with loud or noisy breathing heard at the mouth with the unaided ear. In this study, symptoms, lung function, and chest radiography and bronchoscopic findings were recorded serially before and after 81 cryotherapy sessions in 33 consecutive patients. Most patients improved in terms of overall symptoms, stridor, and haemoptysis and they had an overall improvement in dyspnoea. Relief of dyspnoea was the most common benefit from treatment, the mean improvement in dyspnoea score between the first and the last assessment being 0.5 (p < 0.02).

Stridor had resolved completely in four patients. Four patients had complete resolution of haemoptysis, two after the first treatment and two after the third. In a further two patients haemoptysis improved. In this series, cryotherapy had no effect on cough overall and change in cough score tended not to be sustained. The number of patients with improvement in symptom scores is shown in Table 1.

Table 1. Walsh D.A. ; Maiwand M.O. et al, 1990 Numbers and percentages of patients showing improvement from baseline at the final assessment after cryotherapy

	n	N°	(%) improved
Dyspnoea score	27	10	37
Haemoptysis	9	6	67
Stridor	7	4	56

In other series the only criteria to be regularly reviewed is haemoptysis. Sanderson [7] cites 4 cases of cessation after cryotherapy but without saying how many cases were treated in total. In our series [8] haemoptysis stopped in 80 % of cases. Similar good results have been obtained by Eichler which were reported in the thesis of F.P. Savy [9] with 100 % success rate in a small series. Vergnon has achieved a success rate of 82 % in an unspecified number of cases.

Improvement or disappearance of dyspnoea is variably reported but good results were obtained by Vergnon in 50 % of cases [10] and by Lamy in 42 % [11] (Thesis of C. Rayel-Boisdron).

Improvement of other symptoms is sometimes reported by the same authors with disappearance of wheeze, cough and thoracic pain. In a previous series Maiwand [12] reported an improvement in cough.

Respiratory function has been well reported by Walsh in his study. Whenever possible forced vital capacity (FVC), forced expiratory volume in one second (FEV_1) and maximum expiratory and inspiratory flow rates (MEF, MIF) were recorded from a single forced expiratory and inspiratory deep breath with the Microloop turbine spirometer. After three satisfactory manœuvres the measurements recorded were from the one that gave the highest values for FVC and FEV_1. A 6 minutes walk test was performed at each assessment whenever possible [13]. Arterial blood gases with the patient breathing air at rest were measured initially at the first and fourth assessment. The airway response to 2.5 mg nebulised salbutamol was measured at the first assessment, and at subsequent assessments if the patient showed an improvement initially of 15 % in FEV_1 or FVC after Salbutamol, with an absolute improvement of at least 0.2 (FEV_1) or 0.3 (FVC) l. An increase in MEF or MIF of 20 % of the baseline value, in arterial oxygen tension (PaO_2) of 1 kPa, or in six minutes walk distance of 50 m or a reduction in symptom score of one unit was considered to be an improvement. The number of patients with improvement in lung function after cryotherapy is shown in Table 2. Objective improvement in lung function was seen in 58 % of patients, and the changes in lung function correlated with symptoms.

Table 2. Walsh D.A. ; Maiwand M.O. et al, 1990 Numbers and percentages of patients showing improvement from baseline at the final assessment after cryotherapy

	n	N°	(%) improved
FEV_1	29	7	24
FVC	29	7	24
MEF	29	7	24
MIF	11	3	27
PaO_2	21	7	33
6 minute walk	22	6	27

Guichenez analysed the respiratory function in 10 patients treated before and after cryotherapy. The lesions were located either in the trachea or else the main bronchi, a consistent improvement in spirometry was obtained (see Tables 3 and 4).

Table 3. Average values of FEV_1 and FVC before and after cryotherapy (Guichenez P)

	Before	After
FEV_1	1,810	2,085
FVC	2,850	3,420

These results compare favourably with those found in a published series with laser therapy [14, 15].

Ventilatory and perfusion scintigraphy complete the functional studies. These are being carried out at present.

Radiological results

The effectiveness of cryotherapy is really seen when ventilation of a lung or lobe is compromised. The reventilation of a portion of lung immediately produces an improvement in lung function as well as improvement in symptoms. The area of reventilation may be demonstrated radiologically and the field to be irradiated may be reduced accordingly — this will limit the extent of possible post radiation fibrosis. The benefits of an association between cryotherapy and radiotherapy will be discussed in a later chapter (as the effects of cryotherapy are delayed reventilation rarely occurs immediately after the procedure).

The reventilation may be total (Figs. 4 and 5) or partial (Fig. 6) when the lesion is voluminous and not readily accessible.

Endoscopic results

Benign lesions

These lesions when treated with cryotherapy give very good results. We have seen in a previous chapter that certain tumours are resistant to the effects of cold and that others, such as granulation tissue [16], are very sensitive and give good results with no recurrence months or even years after treatment (Fig. 7). Good results are also obtained when treating myomas or leiomyomas (Fig. 8) even if several sessions of cryotherapy may be necessary. The results are variable with fibrotic stenoses of the bronchus and in cuff like stenoses of the trachea with tracheomalacia cryotherapy is often unsuccessful, however we have obtained some good results (Fig. 9) and Rodgers [2] obtained satisfactory results when treating congenital fibrous stenoses in children using cryotherapy in combination with dissecting forceps. These results are shown in Table 5.

Tumours of low or intermediate malignancy

These tumours are rare and very few have been treated with cryosurgery as they are usually treated surgically.

When surgery is not possible however, treatment with cryotherapy can yield good results.

Table 4. Results of FEV₁ and FVC before and after cryotherapy

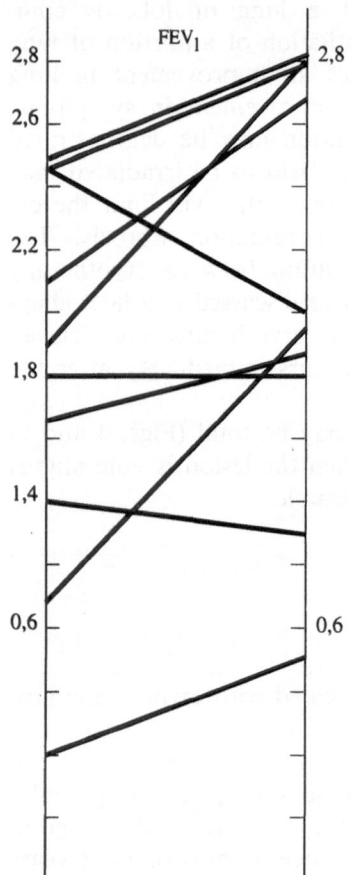

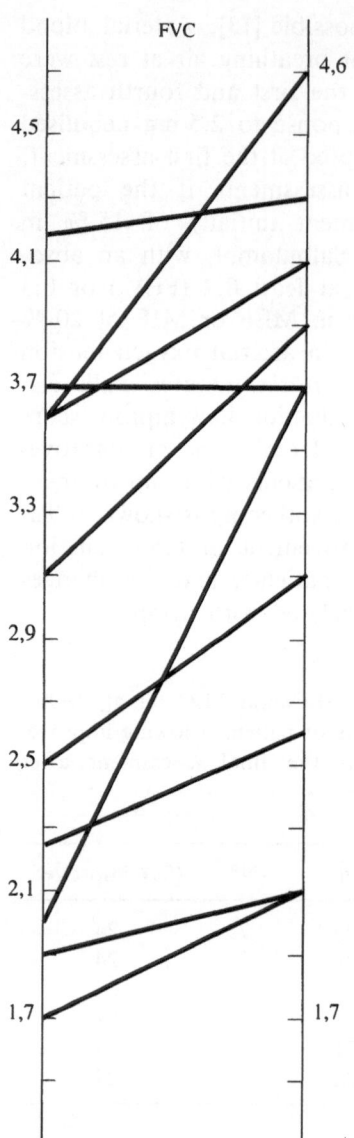

Table 5.

	Authors	Rodgers 1982		Homasson 1986		Eichler 1989		Vergnon 1989		Lamy 1989		Luna Sabate 1990		Roullier 1986	
						Benign lesions									
Histology		n	%	n	%	n	%	n	%	n	%	n	%	n	%
Granulation tissues		4	100	11	95	—	—	2	100	2	100	10	100	1	100
Fibrous stenosis		1	0	2	50	2	0	1	100	—	—	2	50	1	100
Collar shaped stenosis with tracheomalacia		—	—	—	—	—	—	5	0	2	50	—	—	—	—
Lipoma		—	—	1	0	—	—	1	0	—	—	—	—	—	—
Various - Congenital stenosis		8	61	—	—	—	—	—	—	—	—	—	—	—	—
- Aspergilloma		—	—	—	—	1	100	—	—	—	—	—	—	—	—
- Myomas - Leiomyomas		—	—	3	100	—	—	—	—	—	—	—	—	—	—

n = number ; % = percentage of favourable results

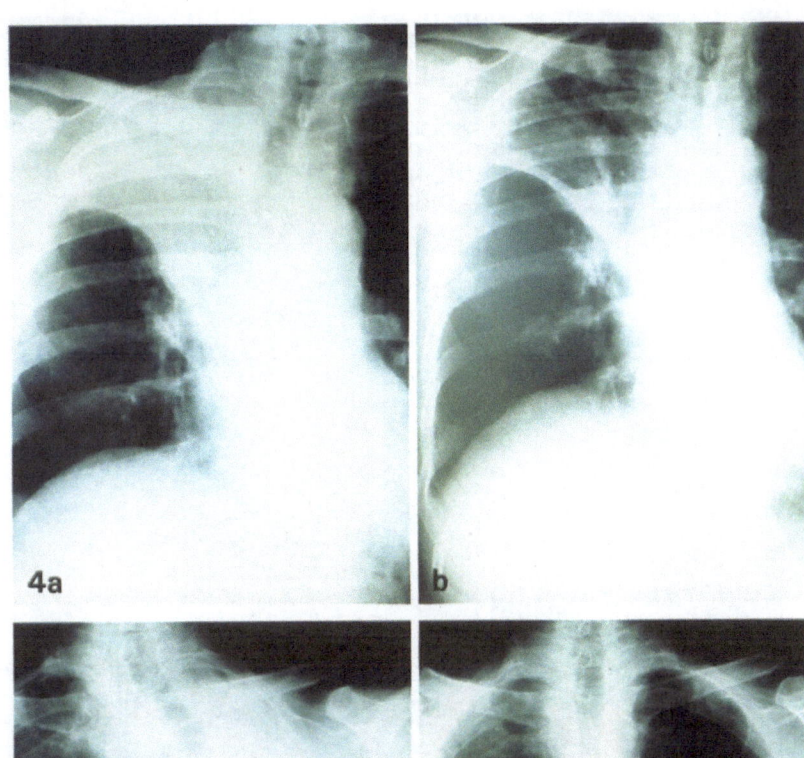

Fig. 4. Total reventilation of right upper lobe

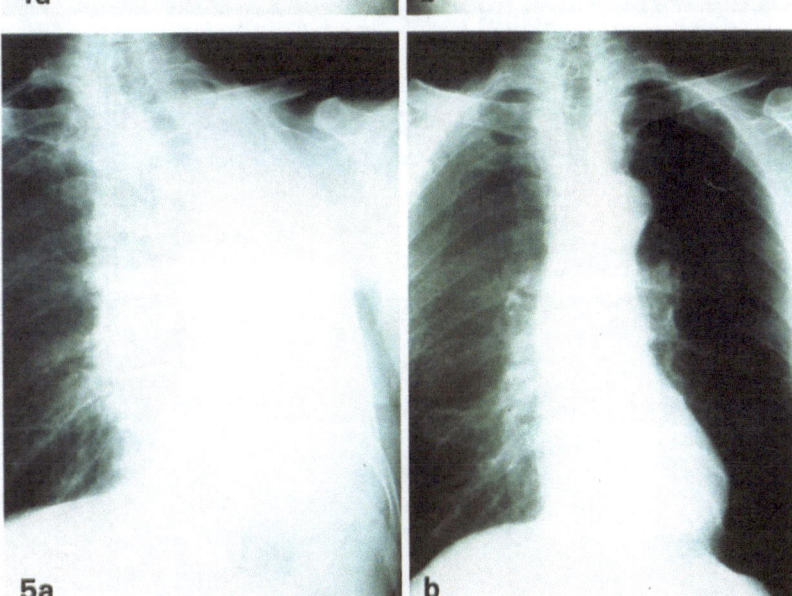

Fig. 5 a, b. Total reventilation of left lung

There have been 11 published cases so far, 6 carcinoids, 3 cylindromas, 1 mucoid squamous cell, and one laryngo-tracheal papilloma. The results are shown in Table 6. The two failures were in carcinoid tumours (Vergnon and Eichler) and were related to technical failures due to the length of the cryoprobe and a faulty probe.

Malignant tumours

Cryotherapy will only destroy the visible endobronchial portion of these tumours and therefore the results are difficult to assess as they depend on various criteria, namely endoscopic appearance and the histology of the tumours. French workers consider that successful treatment may be defined when more than 50 % of the visible tumour is destroyed. Results are considered very good when the relief of obstruction is greater than 80 %. Follow up endoscopies, with biopsies, are carried out with varying frequency depending on the preferences of the workers.

Cryotherapy is thus a palliative treatment in these cases and overall the results are favourable in between 70-80 % of all cases treated according to the criteria used to measure performance.

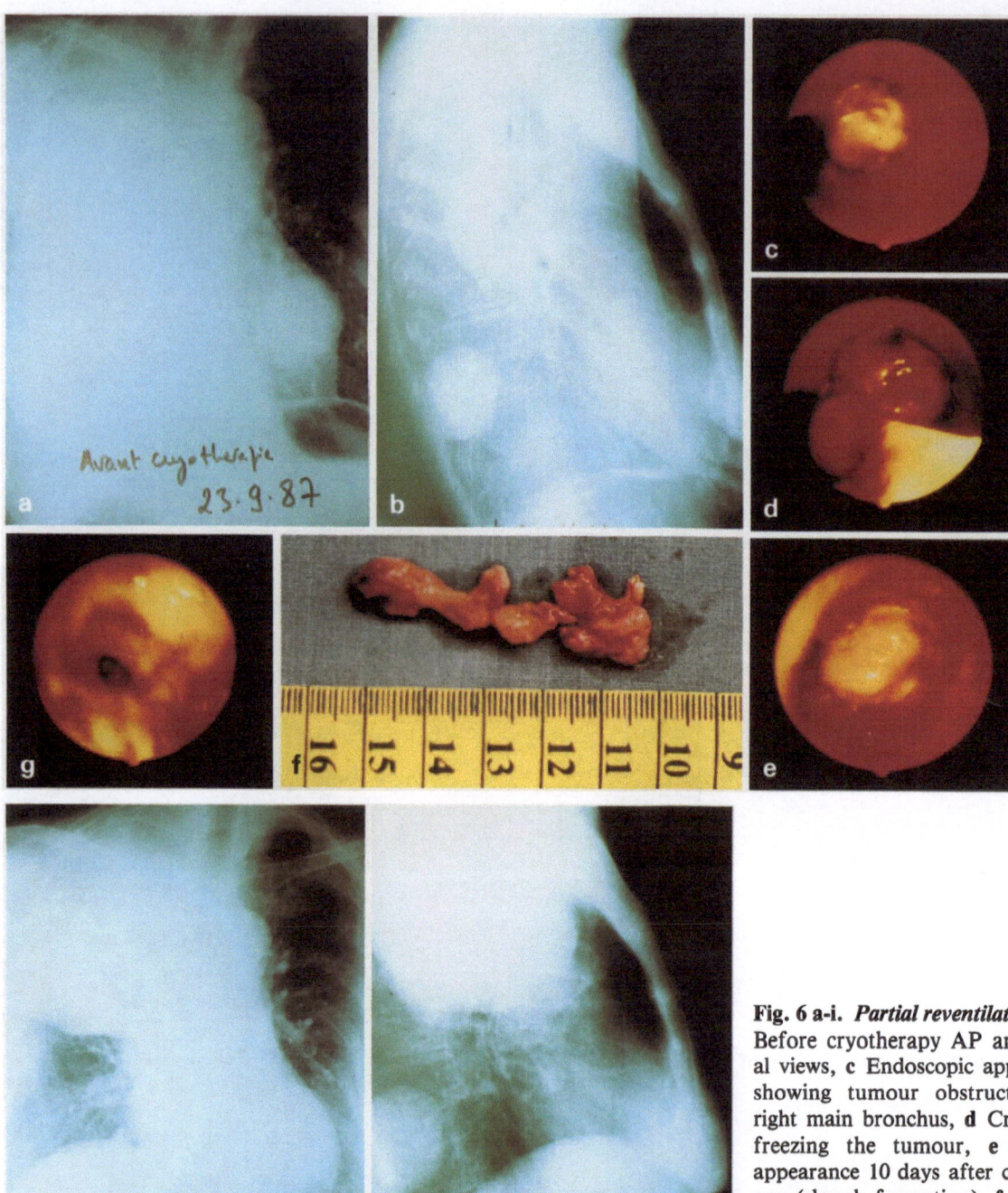

Fig. 6 a-i. *Partial reventilation.* a, b Before cryotherapy AP and lateral views, c Endoscopic appearance showing tumour obstructing the right main bronchus, d Cryoprobe freezing the tumour, e Tumour appearance 10 days after cryotherapy (slough formation), f Slough, g Appearance of bronchus after removal of slough, h, i Radiological appearance showing partial reventilation (AP and lateral views)

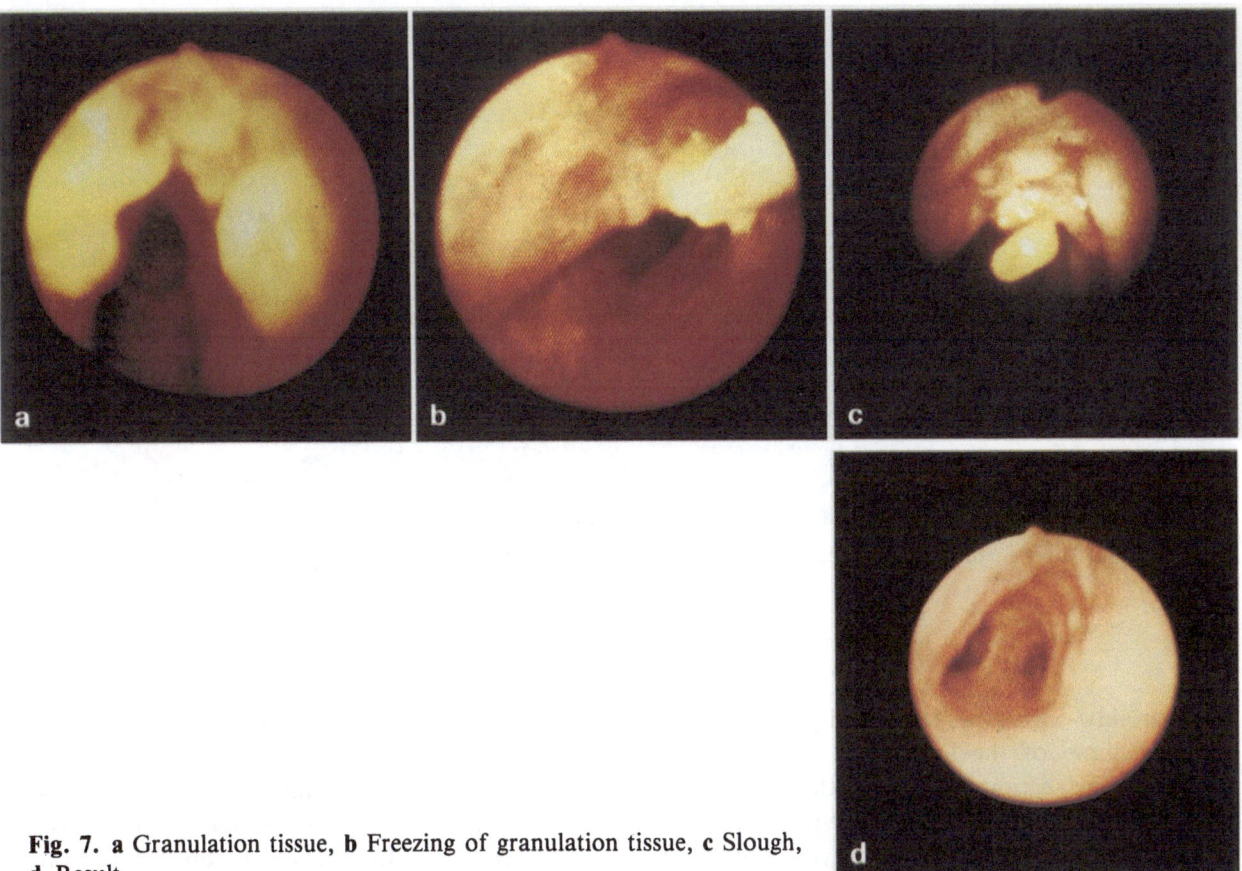

Fig. 7. a Granulation tissue, **b** Freezing of granulation tissue, **c** Slough, **d** Result

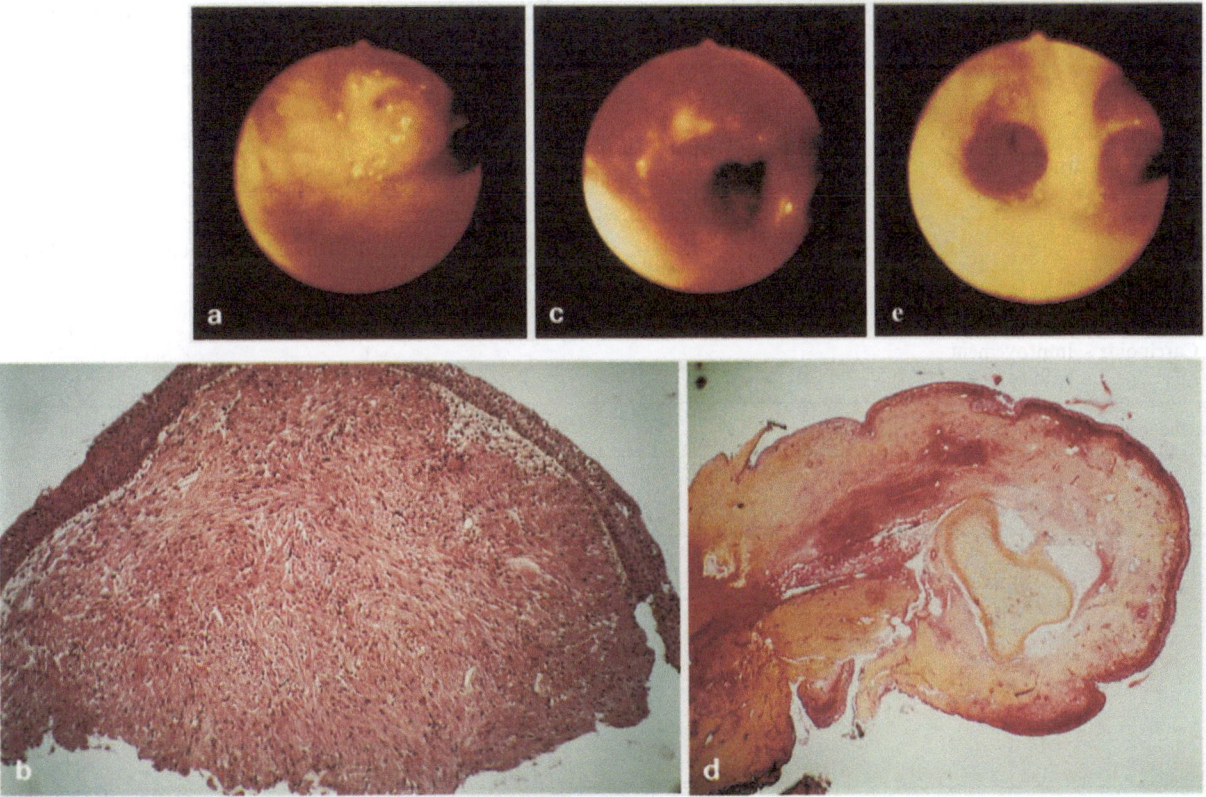

Fig. 8. a Leiomyoma in apical bronchus of right lower lobe, **b** Histological appearance of biopsy, **c** Appearance following slough removal, **d** Histological appearance of slough, **e** Appearance six months after cryotherapy

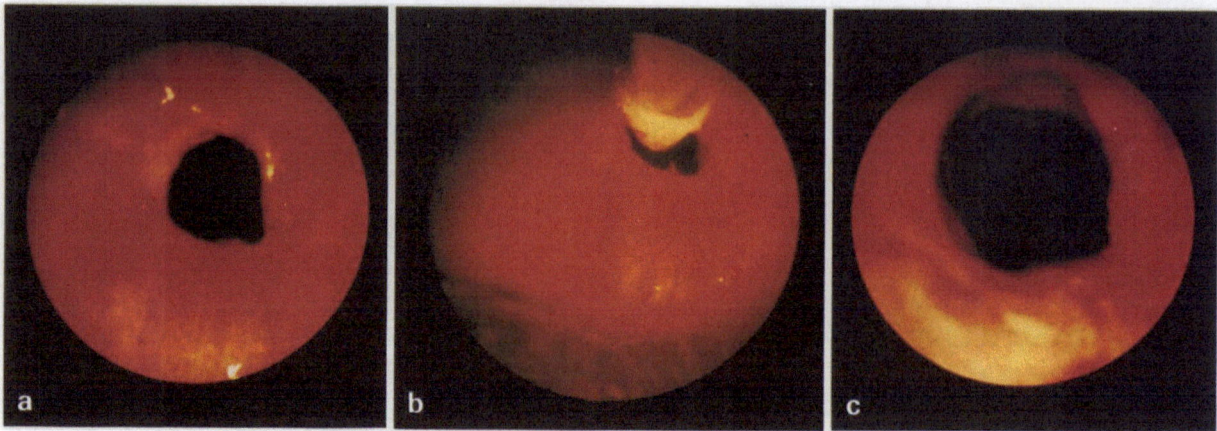

Fig. 9. **a** Cuff-like stenosis of trachea, **b** During cryotherapy, **c** Result

It invariably improves the quality of life by reducing some of the unpleasant symptoms of bronchial obstruction but as yet there has been no significant improvement of survival. The best results have been obtained on polypoid tumours when the cryoprobe may be forced into the tumour to achieve maximal freezing, if possible in the entire tumour. We have included two examples of squamous cell carcinomas treated in this way (Figs. 10 and 11).

Cryotherapy has its limits however and when a tumour is very large or rapidly growing the results are poor. In tracheal lesions, if the obstruction is equal to or greater than 50 % of the airway we consider cryotherapy to be contraindicated, however the oedema produced follow-

Table 6. Tumours with reduced malignancy

Histology / Authors	Sanderson 1981	Eichler 1988	Vergnon 1989	Homasson Baud 1990	Luna Sabate 1990	Tolstuchow 1990
Carcinoids - Success				1	1	1
Carcinoids - Improvement				1		
Carcinoids - Failure		1	1			
Mucco-epidermoid tumours				1 success		
Cylindroma - Success	1		1			
Cylindroma - Failure			1			
Papilloma					1 success	

Fig. 10. **a** Radiological appearance showing collapse of right upper lobe, **b** Squamous cell carcinoma obstructing the right upper lobe bronchus, **c** Tumour being frozen, **d** Appearance immediately following freezing, **e** Radiological appearance showing reventilation, **f** Follow up endoscopy ten days later showing small slough ▶

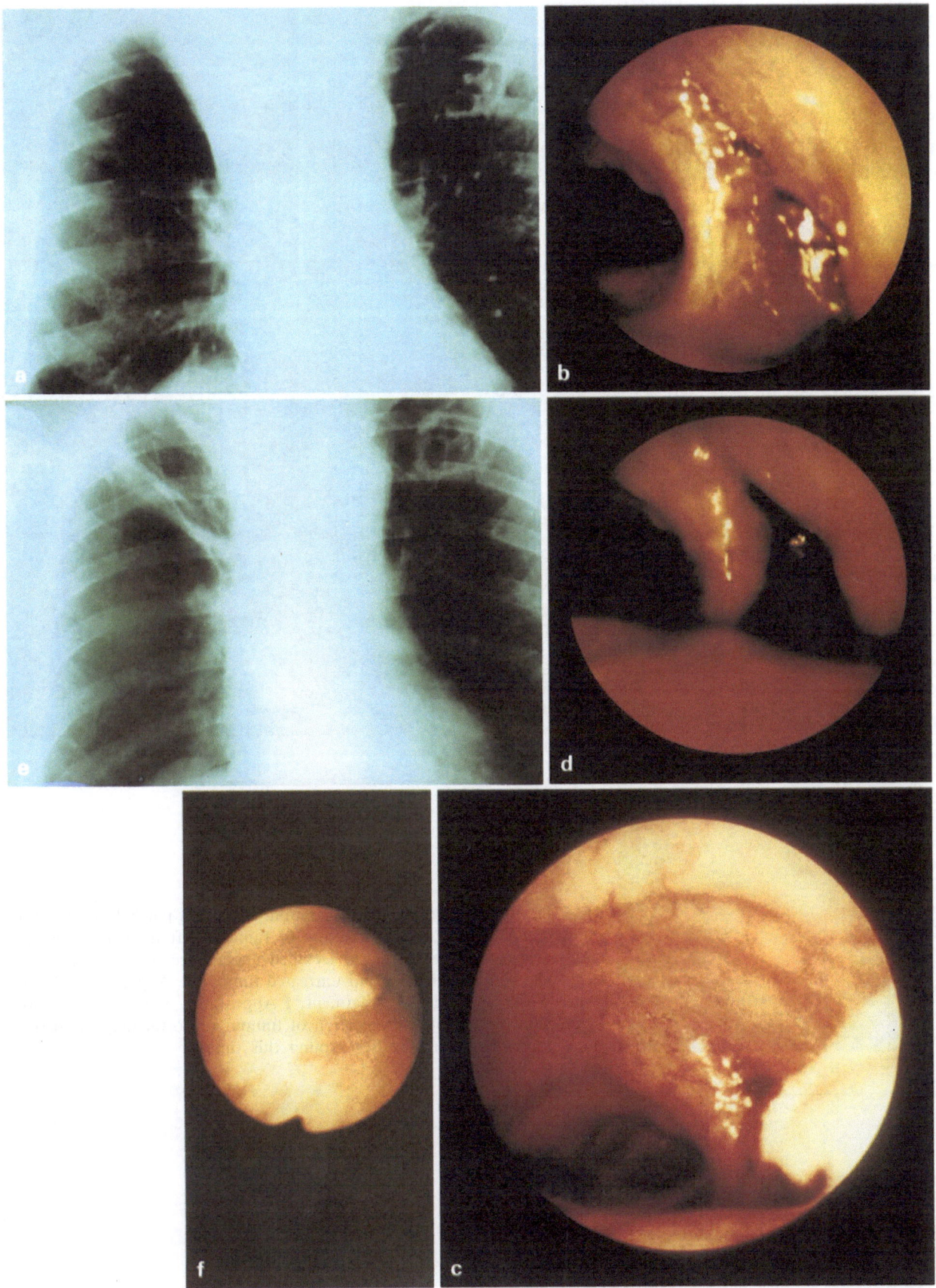

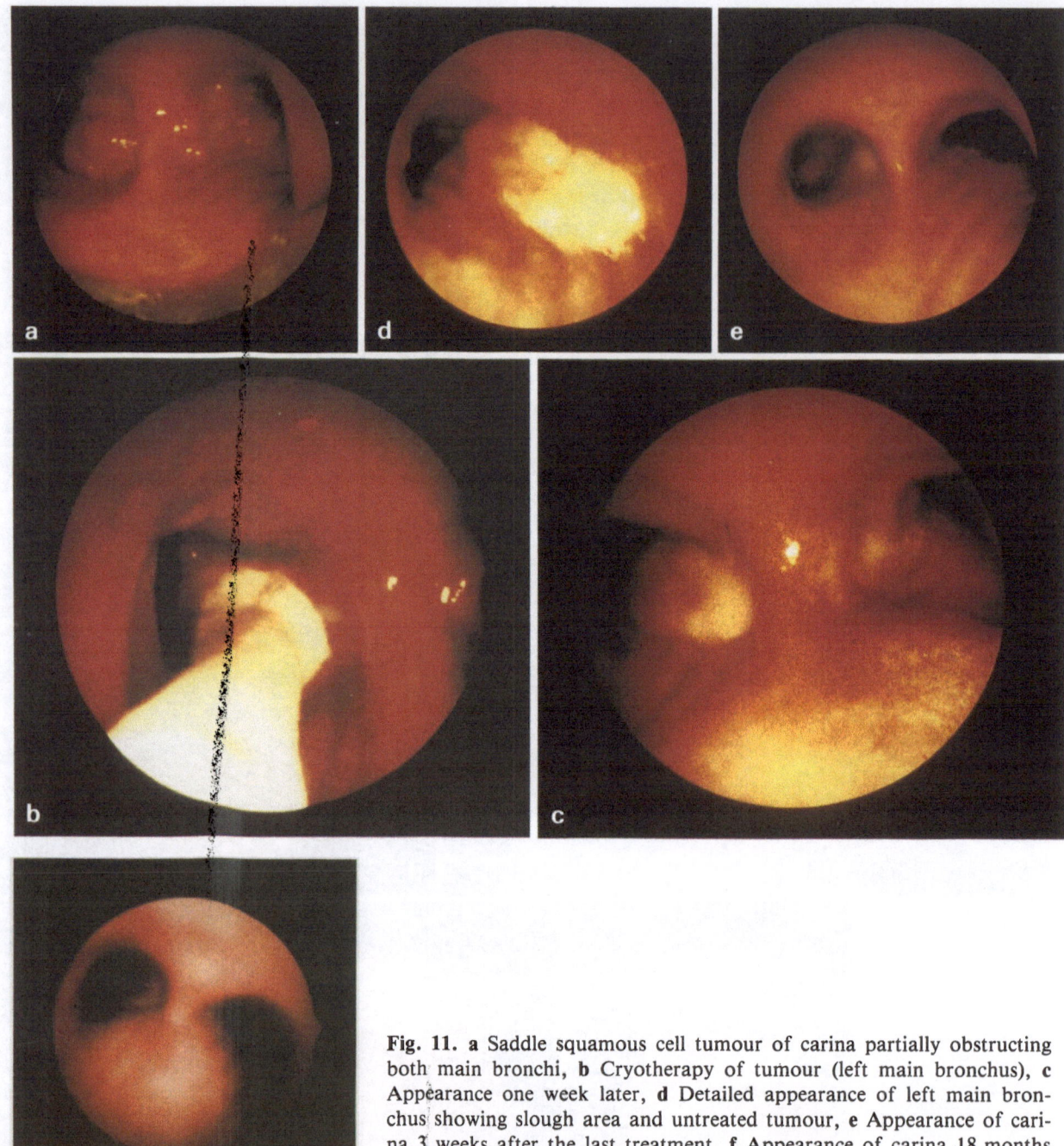

Fig. 11. a Saddle squamous cell tumour of carina partially obstructing both main bronchi, **b** Cryotherapy of tumour (left main bronchus), **c** Appearance one week later, **d** Detailed appearance of left main bronchus showing slough area and untreated tumour, **e** Appearance of carina 3 weeks after the last treatment, **f** Appearance of carina 18 months later showing complete eradication of tumour (unfortunately the patient died from distant metastases around this time)

ing therapy does not exceed the volume of tumour initially treated. In our series [8-17] we did not have any problems with local œdema ; the control chest x-ray both 2 and 24 hours following treatment did not show any significant changes or aggravated ventilatory problems. We think that the cartilaginous armature of the tracheobronchial tree helps to maintain airway potency.

With practice and careful patient selection all workers have found an improvement in results. For Maiwand [18] the best results were obtained in tracheal tumours as these lesions are easily accessible to a rigid bronchoscope and the more powerful rigid or semi-stiff cryoprobes may be used. Savy [8] also obtained good results in 90 % of cases when treating tracheal lesions using semirigid or flexible cryoprobes. Guichenez [9] found that not all tumours of the left main bronchus were accessible to a rigid bronchoscope which led to certain failures, mainly due to technical reasons and in his series there were twice as many failures than successes which demonstrates that the results partially depends on the site and accessibility of the lesions.

Table 7 includes the results of malignant tumours treated in the most important series carried out in the States and Europe (France, Great Britain, Spain and Czechoslovakia).

Table 7. Results — Malignant tumours

Authors	Year	Number of patients	Favourable results %
Sanderson	1981	28	54
Homasson	1986	22	59
	1990	195	72
Maiwand	1987	130	76
Walsh	1990	33	77
Eichler Savy	1988	52	65
Vergnon Guichenez	1989	40	55
Lamy Rayel-Boisdron	1989	40	55
Luna Sabate	1990	12	80
Pesek	1990	26	76

References

1. Walsh DA, Maiwand MO, Nath AR, Lockwood P, Lloyd MH, Saab M (1990) Bronchoscopic cryotherapy for advanced bronchial carcinoma. Thorax 45 : 509-513
2. Pesek M, Simecek C, Bruha F (1990) Kryokoagulation in der Behandlung von Bronchialtumoren. Z Erkrank Atm Org 175 : 126-131
3. Rodgers BM, Moazam F, Talbert JL (1983) Endotracheal cryotherapy in the treatment of refractory airway strictures. Ann Thor Surg 35 : 52-57
4. Roden S, Homasson JP (1989) Une nouvelle indication de la cryothérapie endobronchique : l'extraction de corps étrangers. Presse Med 18 : 897
5. Ozenne G, Vergnon JM, Roullier A, Blanc-Jouvan F, Courty G (1990) Cryotherapy of *in situ* or micro invasive bronchial carcinoma. Chest 98 (suppl) : 105
6. Medical Research Council (1966) Questionnaire on respiratory symptoms. London : Medical Research Council
7. Sanderson DR, Neel HB, Fontana S (1981) Bronchoscopic cryotherapy. Ann Otol 90 : 354-358
8. Homasson JP, Renault P, Angebault M, Bonniot JP, Bell NJ (1986) Bronchoscopic cryotherapy for airway strictures caused by tumors. Chest 90 : 159-164
9. Savy FP (1988) Cryothérapie bronchique. Effets du traitement endoscopique de 111 lésions bronchiques par cryothérapie à l'aide de sondes souples ou semirigides. Thesis. Limoges University, France
10. Guichenez P (1989) Expérience de 3 ans de la cryothérapie endobronchique par sonde semi-rigide. A propos de 107 traitements. Thesis. Saint-Étienne University, France
11. Rayel-Boisdron C (1989) La cryothérapie en pathologie trachéo-bronchique. Thesis. Nancy University, France
12. Maiwand MO (1987) Cryotherapy for advanced carcinoma of bronchi and trachea. Cryotherapy 9 : 22-24
13. Butland RJA, Pang J, Gross ER, Woodlock AA, Geddes DM (1982) Two, six, and 12 minutes walking test in respiratory disease. Br Med J 284 : 1607-1608
14. Gelb AF, Epstein JD (1984) Laser treatment of lung cancer. Chest 86 : 662-666
15. Brutinel WM, Cortese DA, McDougall JC, Gillio RG, Bergstrath EJ (1987) A two year experience with neodymium. YAG laser in endobronchial obstruction. Chest 91 : 159-165
16. Bonniot JP, Angebault M, Roullier A, Homasson JP (1986) Traitement des granulomes trachéobronchiques par cryothérapie. Presse Med 15 : 667
17. Homasson JP, Angebault M, Bonniot JP, Baud D, Roden S, François-Coudray S (1990) Cryotherapy of benign and malignant tracheo-bronchial tumors — Report of 250 cases. Chest 98 : 131
18. Maiwand MO (1986) Cryotherapy for advanced carcinoma of the trachea and bronchi. Br Med J 293 : 181-182

Histopathology

Jean-Paul Homasson and Françoise Lange

Experimental findings using the cryomicroscope

Cryodestruction may be studied histologically. In the chapter « The process of freezing and the mechanism of damage during cryosurgery » Rubinsky describes the cryomicroscope which allows the study of the effect of ice formation both intra and extracellularly during the freezing process [1].

The cryomicroscope system used for our study is equipped with a programmable freezing and thawing stage [2]. The temperature of the sample is measured by a copper-constantan thermocouple and the accuracy of the system is ± 0.2° C. Temperature and time are displayed during freezing and thawing and optically superimposed onto the images. With a prism, it is possible to photograph with a 400 ASA black and white film and simultaneously to make a video recording on an Umatic system.

Cell behaviour is observed in bright field observation, phase contrast or using Nomarski optics.

Drops of cell suspensions (about 5 μl) are placed between two glass slides for the observation and subjected to a freeze-thaw cycle under the microscope. The sample may be cooled or warmed through the temperature range of about + 40 to − 180° C (with the use of liquid nitrogen), at any rate between 0, 1 and 60° C/minute.

With this cryomicroscope we have observed cancerous bronchial cells either isolated or else in tissue (Fig. 1). It has been possible to study the initial effect of cold which corresponds to a mechanical distortion [3]. The extracellular freezing starts with finger like structures (Fig. 2) these compress and deform the cells — « the pack ice effect » and then interfere with the ionic exchanges across the membranes. Intracellular freezing, which is very traumatic, occurs secondarily and in a sudden flash. The cells have been cooled to − 40° C (the temperature reached in a few seconds in the ball of ice which is in contact with the cryoprobe). A eutectic freezing state is achieved (Fig. 3). On thawing the cells are distorted (Fig. 4) — the nucleoles have disappeared and the cell membranes torn.

With the aid of video cassette recordings we have been able to observe the intracellular freezing frame by frame at 1/25th of a second intervals. Figure 5 shows a group of cancerous bronchial cells (squamous cell carcinoma). The freezing front surrounds the cell and one can clearly see ice crystals appearing intracellularly whilst adjacent cells remain unfrozen.

Another study, in collaboration with J.-P. Thiery (National Centre of Scientific Research, Cell Biology Centre, Ivry, France) allowed us to look at the different levels of cellular distortion which occur within the ice ball surrounding a cryoprobe. In this experiment we froze a sample of ascitic fluid containing cells from a rat with ascitic hepatoma (Zajdela strain) using a bronchial cryoprobe. At the same time we studied the survival of these cells after freezing, by reinjecting them into the peritoneal cavity of a rat. The area in contact with the cryoprobe reaches a temperature of − 40° C almost immediately and the cells are completely destroyed. However at the edge of the ice ball

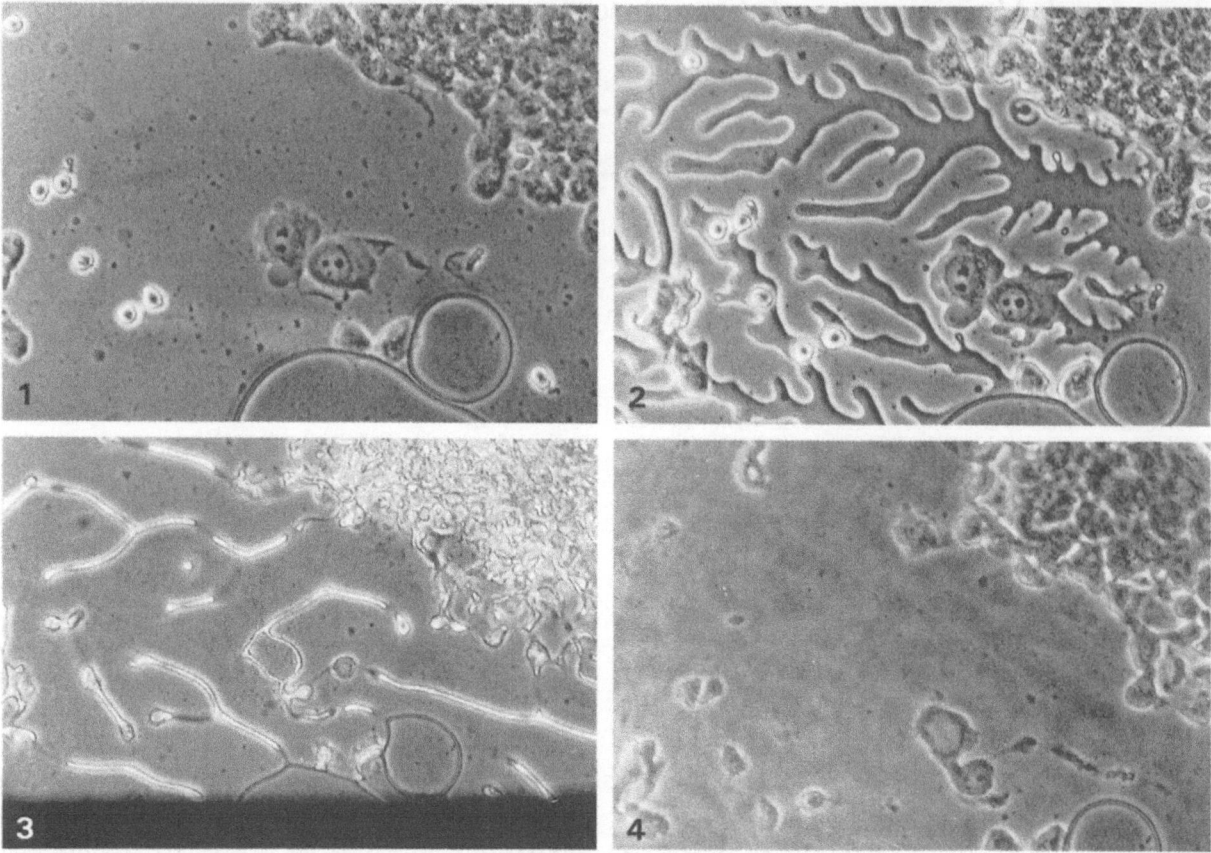

Fig. 1. Squamous cell carcinoma (size : 30μm approx M × 125)

Fig. 2. Finger-like structures

Fig. 3. Eutectic freezing

Fig. 4. Appearance of cells on thawing (after only one freeze-thaw cycle)

the cellular structures are preserved. There is thus a gradient of destruction as shown in Figure 6. The direct action of freezing is compounded by a cryothrombosis which leads to tissue necrosis.

Cryotherapy and bronchus

The histopathological studies were carried out in order to verify the correlation between the clinical results obtained with this technique and the consequences on the tissue. In order to do this all samples were treated by the same method. The biopsies to be studied histologically were fixed in Bouin's liquid then set in paraffin before being cut and stained by haematoxylin/eosin/safran (HES). At the same time the samples to undergo study of their ultra structure were immediately fixed in 2.5 % glutaraldehyde at

pH 7.45 and stored in a cool place. They underwent further fixation in 1 % osmium tetroxide. Following this they were incorporated in epon. A few slices were taken from each block and stained with Toluidine blue — these served as markers for the ultra thin slices. The main part of our material consisted of carcinomas, usually squamous cell carcinomas, and a few benign tumours. We also studied the effect of cryotherapy on normal bronchial epithelium. From the outset it must be stated that the histological appearance and the ultrastructure varied according to the number of freeze-thaw cycles and also from zone to zone within the same biopsy sample.

The part played by the number of freeze-thaw cycles in the destruction of cells is particularly well seen if a biopsy of a slough is examined 8-10 days after cryotherapy for an obstructed

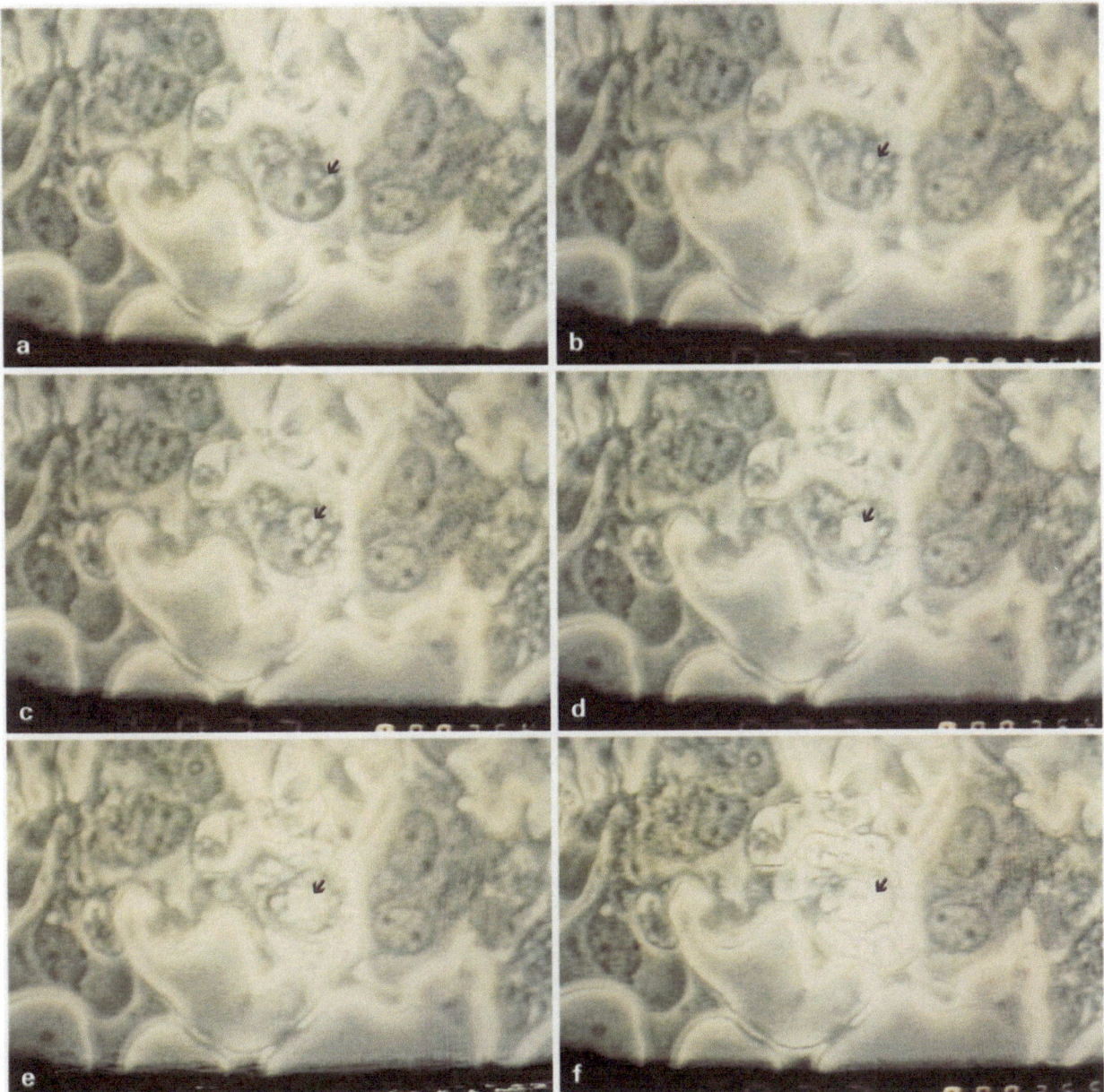

Fig. 5 a-f. Squamous cell carcinoma. Magnification × 125. Intracellular freezing appearing in a flash. The images occur at intervals of 1/25th of a second. Appearance of intracelllar ice crystals *(arrow)*

bronchial lumen. Histologically it consists of acidophilic material containing outlines of cells or nuclear debris which are difficult to identify (Fig. 7). Under electron microscopy all that is seen is cellular debris with hardly any identifiable structures. Fragments of basement membrane and fibrin are all that are left in a squamous cell carcinoma treated with several cycles of cryotherapy (Fig. 8). This necrosis is particularly well seen in conjunctival tumours which need 8-10 freeze-

thaw cycles. Ultra structure examination reveals necrotic debris with a few cell fragments (Fig. 9).

Infiltrating epithelial tumours however yield slightly more heterogenous results. A single freeze-thaw cycle is all that is required in order to obtain a biopsy specimen and the cell structures are easily recognizable such that tumour typing is possible. In this way a squamous cell carcinoma is readily identifiable due to the large cells and the surrounding structures. Diagnosis

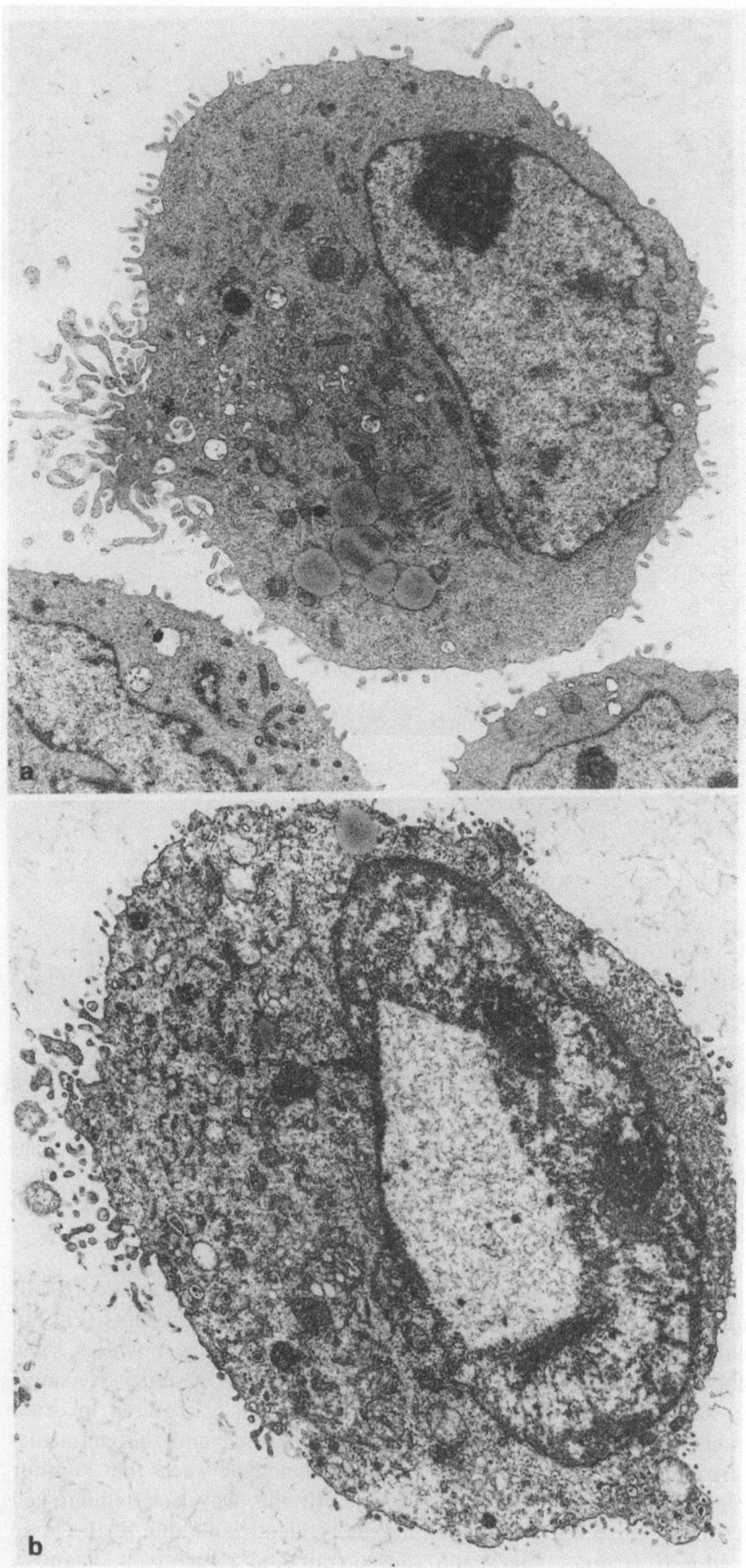

Fig. 6. a Tumour cell (Ascitic hepatoma — Zajdela Strain) in a non frozen suspension (magnification 455 × 13 500) **b** Cell from central zone (zone a) showing nucleus with large crystal and oedematous cytoplasm with numerous swollen mitochondria and distorted microvilli (magnification 525 × 13 500), **c** Cells from periphery (zone b) with varying degrees of damage (x = viable cell y = non viable cell) (magnification 905 × 9 000)

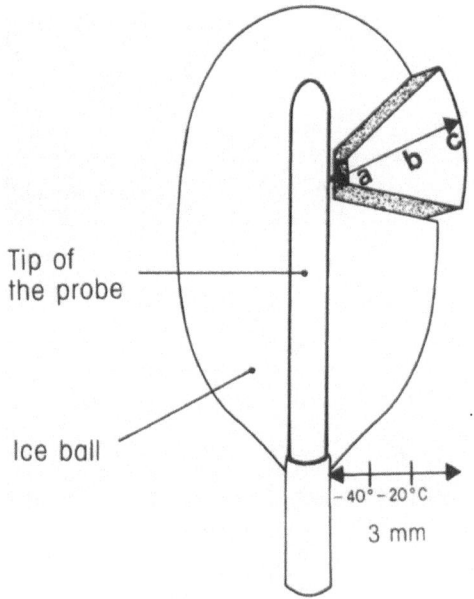

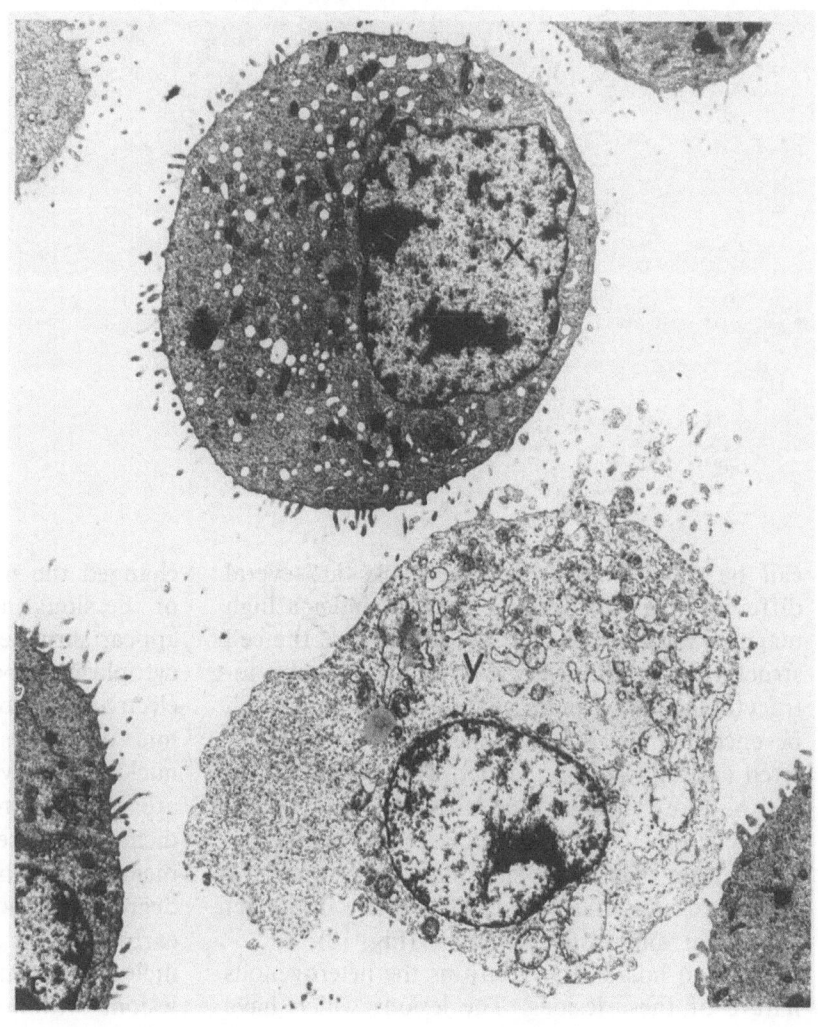

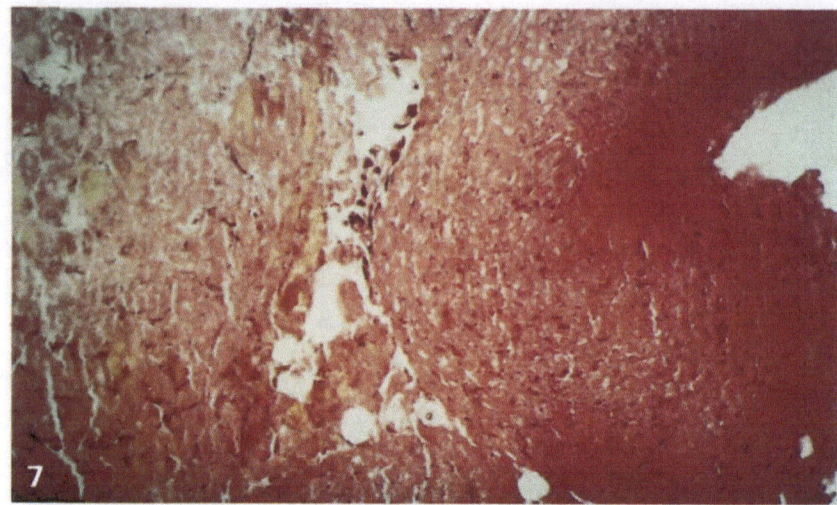

Fig. 7. Acidophilic slough. HES × 250

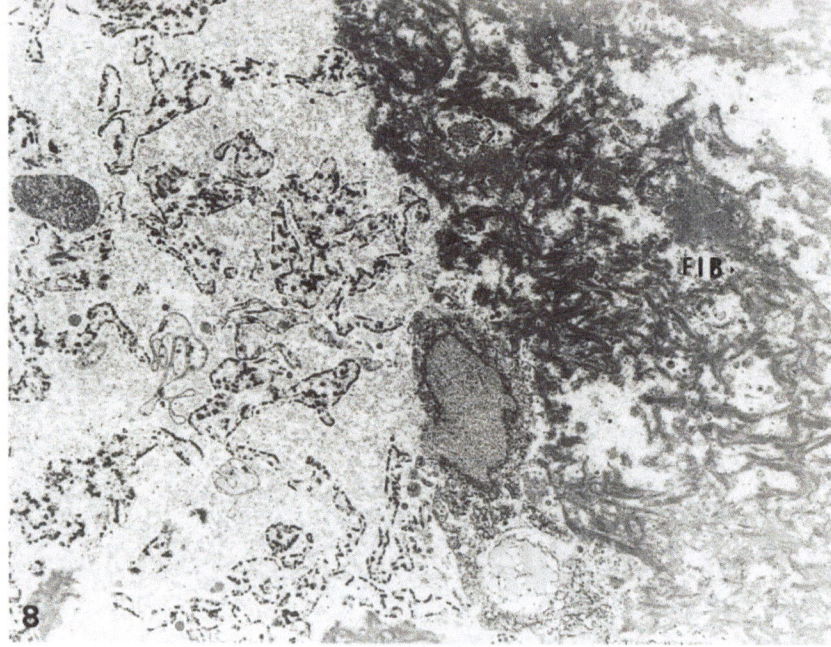

Fig. 8. Bronchus (E.M. ± × 4,500). Cellular fragments of a squamous cell carcinoma with fibrin (FIB)

can be reliably made. If one looks at several different areas of the same tumour under a high magnification one would see areas where the cell structure was less well preserved in particular intracytoplasmic vacuoles and shrunken nuclei will be encountered. The cytoplasm may also be altered and appear less distinct. These appearances will be more marked if a fairly thick cut of the biopsy is taken, there will be areas where the tissues are well preserved and other areas where the cells are manifestly altered with indistinct cytoplasm and distorted nuclei (Fig. 10).

Electron microscopy confirms the heterogenous nature of these lesions. The lesions which have changed the most (outside the massive necrosis of the slough area) indicate cell death. The cells appear shrunken having lost their cohesion. Their cytoplasm appears dark as it is very dense and electrons cannot pass (Fig. 11). The intracytoplasmic organelles are no longer visible and the nucleoli are severely pycnotic or absent. There are areas which are less changed but which also indicate severe cellular damage — distortion of cell membranes which are broken in places, varying degrees of vacuolisation of the cytoplasm and early pycnotic nuclei (Fig. 12). When the biopsy includes the margin of the tumour one can see lesions within the bronchial mucosa. The cyto-

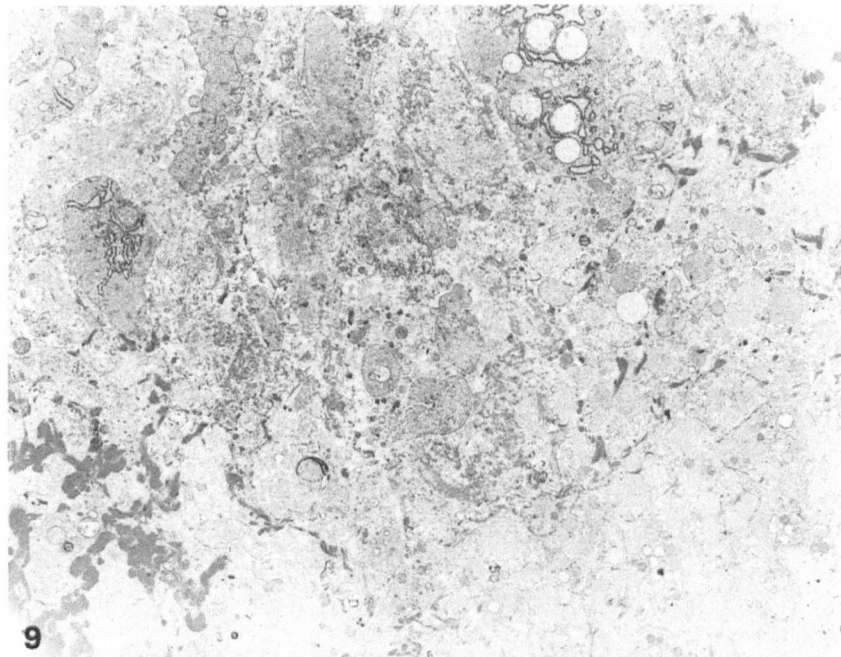

Fig. 9. Bronchus (E.M. × 4,500). Benign muscular tumour treated with cryotherapy

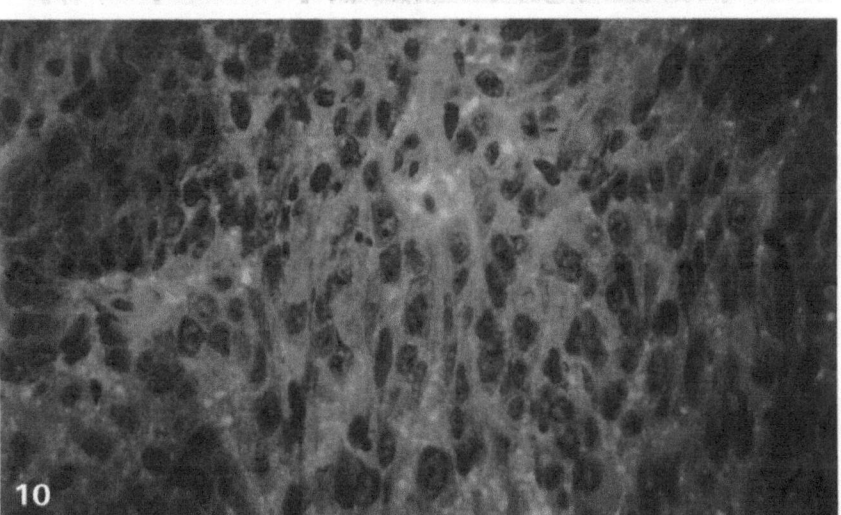

Fig. 10. Cell changes in a thin section. (Toluidine − blue stain × 250)

plasm of endothelial cells and some fibroblasts appear either very dark or else with vacuoles of varying sizes (Fig. 13).

We think that the heterogenous nature of these lesions may be explained by the number of freeze-thaw cycles, the distance of the tissue studied from the point of application of the cryoprobe and the nature of the tissues studied.

As well as the changes observed in tumour tissue treated by cryotherapy, the effect of cold has specific effects on normal bronchial mucosa and these changes were encountered in the three cases that we studied.

The biopsies were taken when cryotherapy was

being used to achieve haemostasis. The histological appearance under light microscope revealed characteristic respiratory epithelium. Under electron microscopy alongside fragments of normal epithelium were areas with specific changes. There was obvious evidence of cellular damage : intracytoplasmic vacuoles ; pycnotic nuclei and distortions of basement membranes (Fig. 14). These changes were similar to those already described. However we also noted a specific change to the cilia. The cells had lost their cilia which appeared severed at their basal body which corresponds to their point of implantation in the cell (Fig. 15). These changes are specific and to our knowledge

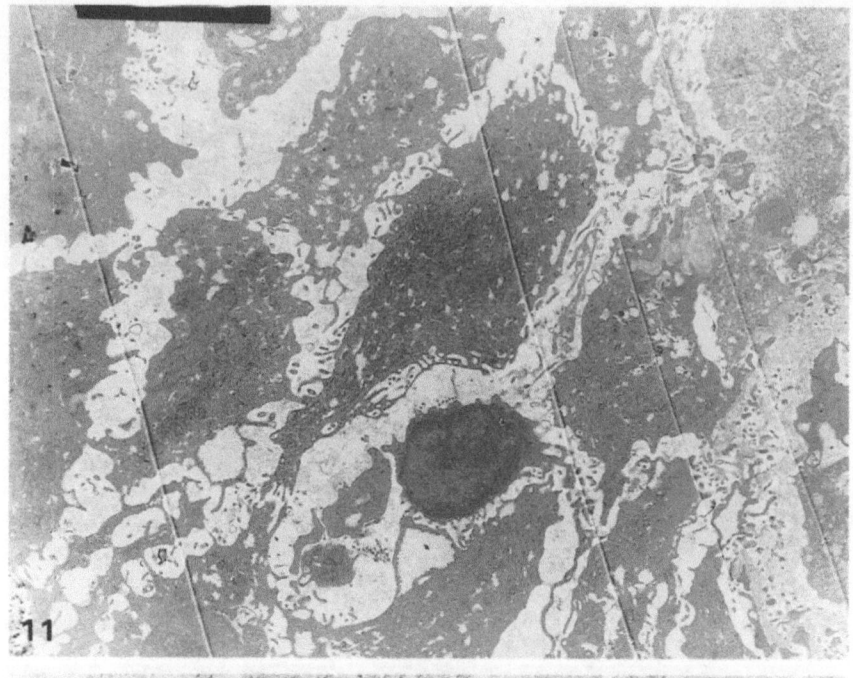

Fig. 11. Shrinkage and condensation of tumour cells after cryotherapy (E.M. × 3,300)

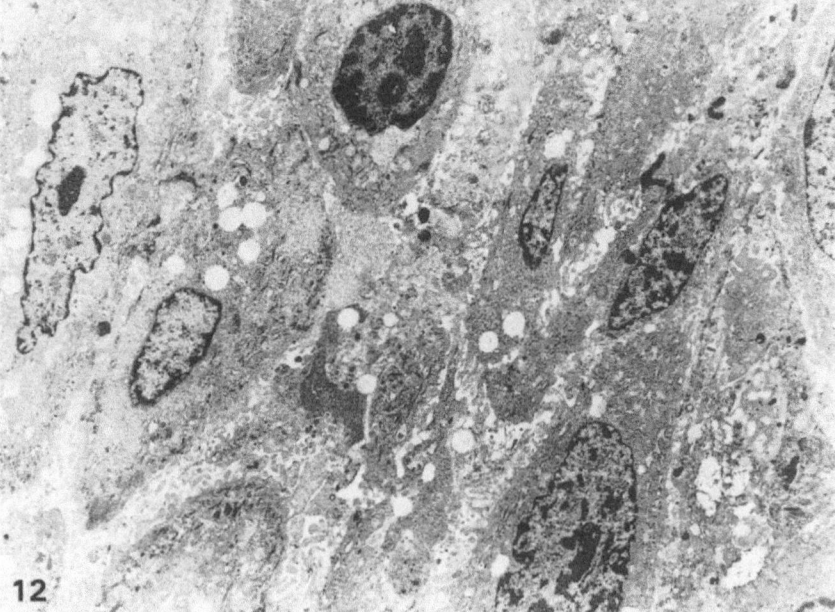

Fig. 12. Several cells showing vacuoles in cytoplasm (E.M. × 3,900)

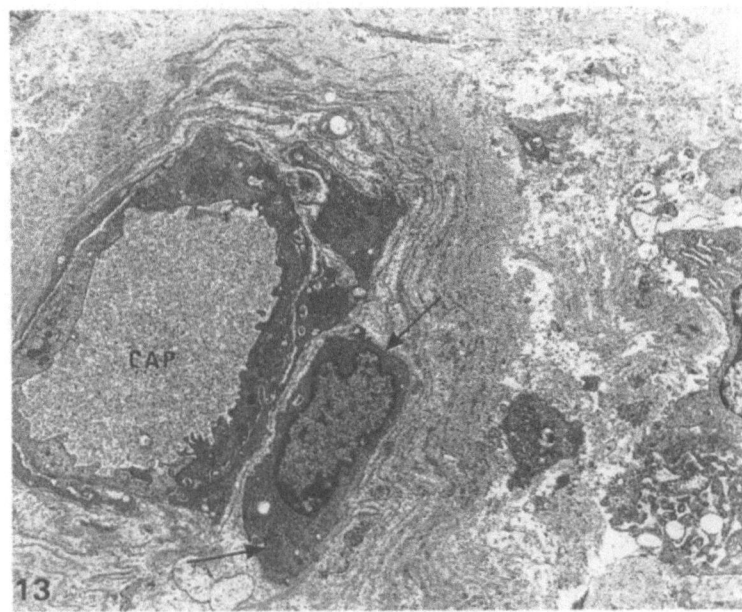

Fig. 13. Cytoplasm of capillary epithelial (CAP) and fibroblast (∕) cells showing increased density (E.M. × 3,900)

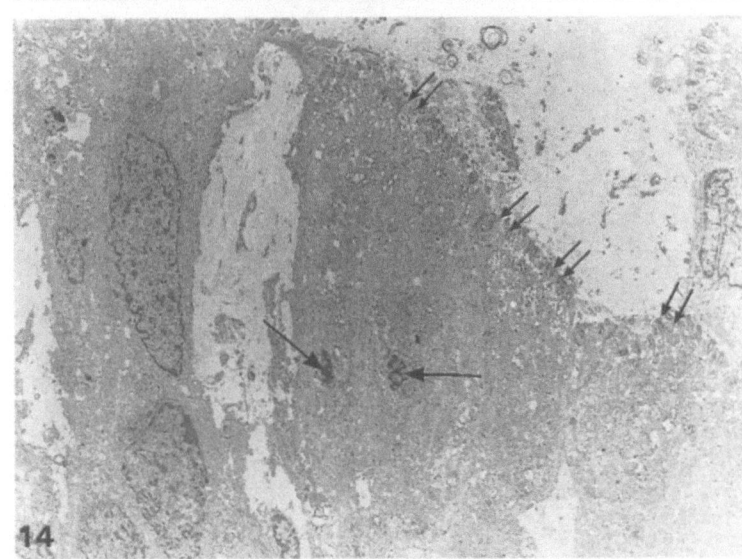

Fig. 14. Bronchus showing necrotic cells with pycnotic nuclei (∕) and widespread decapitation of cilia (∕∕) (E.M. × 3,300)

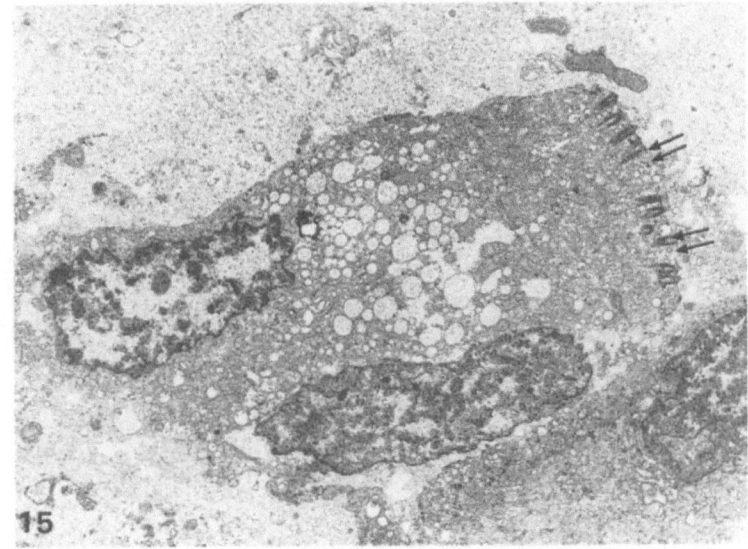

Fig. 15. Bronchus showing cells with vacuoles in cytoplasm and absence of cilia (∕∕) (E.M. 9,100)

have not been described in any other study of ciliary epithelium.

In conclusion, cryotherapy, as well as achieving biopsies of sufficient quality to allow accurate diagnosis causes significant tissue damage to both epithelial and fibroblastic cells. This damage can vary from simple cytoplasmic vacuoles to complete disparition of the tissue architecture. The degree of damage depends on the number of freeze-thaw cycles as well as other factors not fully explained.

Acknowledgements. We thank M. Jondet who allowed us to use his cryomicroscope at the Research Foundation of Hormones in Paris and J.-P. Thiery with whom we collaborated in these studies.

References

1. Rubinsky B, Ikeda M (1985) A cryomicroscope using directional solidification for the controlled freezing of biological materials. Cryobiology 22 : 55-68
2. Jondet M, Dominique S, Scholler R (1984) Effects of freezing and thawing on mammalian oocyte. Cryobiology 21 : 192-199
3. Homasson JP (1990) Cryothérapie en pneumologie. Revue des données fondamentales et cliniques. Rev Pneumol Clin 46 : 189-193

Technical failures or short-comings of the equipment

Jean-Paul Homasson

Contraindications

Cryotherapy is a safe technique and there are practically no contraindications to its use. The real contraindications are those of the endoscopy and or anaesthetic. Patients with cancer are frequently in a poor general state often with a fairly mediocre respiratory function. It is therefore necessary to make a preliminary assessment of the benefits a patient could obtain from cryotherapy and not to submit them to a general anaesthetic and bronchoscopy which could be dangerous.

The main and possibly only contraindication to the technique is in asphyxiating stenoses when the tracheal obstruction is equal to or greater than 50 %. Acute respiratory distress is an emergency. Cryotherapy has a delayed effect. These patients must be treated with a laser first even if subsequent treatment with cryotherapy is used during the same procedure.

Cryotherapy should not be considered for uncontrolled haemorrhage or indeed for secondary haemorrhage from a lesion which is inaccessible to an endoscope.

We also believe that cryotherapy is contraindicated in cases of extrinsic compression. However, Maiwand has treated such lesions [1] but with results considerably less good than for those obtained in relieving endobronchial obstructions (Table 1).

Oesophageal carcinoma with posterior tracheal invasion where there is an absence of tracheal cartilage is another instance where care should be taken. Lamy in the thesis of Rayel-Boisdron [2] reported a case of a tracheo oesophageal fistula following the extraction of an enormous polypoid tumour treated by cryodestruction.

In voluminous tumours cryotherapy is not beneficial.

Complications

One major benefit of cryotherapy is that it is harmless.

Some problems have been signalled by all authors but they have always been minor problems. In our experience [3] a few patients had a mild fever the same evening, but this may occur after any bronchial endoscopy.

A tachycardia often appears during bronchial endoscopy and it is prudent to have electrocardiographic monitoring throughout the examination. ECG monitoring revealed the cause of death of one elderly woman : major myocardial ischaemia at intubation, which was a consequence of the bronchoscopy. Occasionally one sees a bradycardia during freezing in lesions situated in the left main bronchus.

Table 1. Effect of cryotherapy on obstructions (Maiwand M.O.)

Principal obstruction	Patients affected before treatment	Patients improved after treatment
Intraluminal	77	71
Extraluminal	26	8

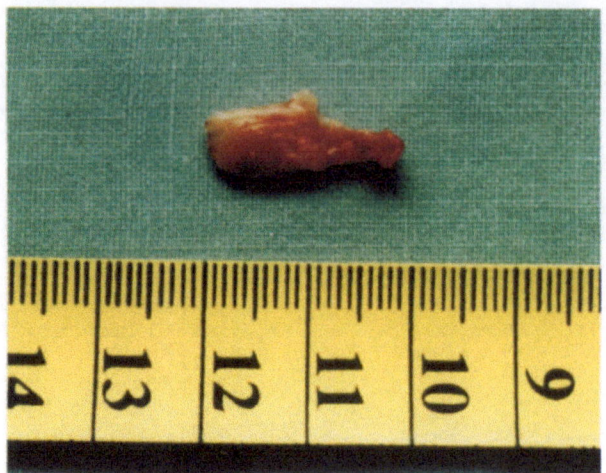

Fig. 1. Slough

After cryotherapy, a necrotic slough will form in the bronchial tree ; no haemoptysis occurs. With a cough, this slough could fall into another bronchus and might be responsible for ventilatory disturbance. Therefore, endoscopy is carried out one week to ten days following cryotherapy to aspirate this slough (Fig. 1).

Freezing has a haemostatic effect and haemoptysis due to a lesion visible endoscopically may be an indication for cryotherapy. However, the haemoptysis may persist and even increase during the 24 hours following treatment. Vergnon in the thesis of Guichenez [4] reported only one case of severe haemorrhage during 107 procedures.

A cough is sometimes reported possibly related to the irritation of intubation. A transitory increase in dyspnoea has also been reported several times. A. Roullier [5] in the thesis of Farlet [6] reported a single case of anaemia due to cold agglutins as a result of freezing.

Early death occurring within the week following cryotherapy has not been attributed directly to the procedure except in two cases, one by Vergnon in a series of 66 patients and the other by Lamy in a series of 44 patients. Both patients had very haemorrhagic tumours and they died from a catastrophic haemoptysis 5 and 8 days following cryotherapy which could have been the cause.

Technical failures or weaknesses in the equipment

Technical failures may be linked to the rigid bronchoscope. They occur essentially when the lesions are situated in the left main bronchus with pulmonary collapse and consequent distortion of the angle of the bronchus or else in the upper lobes sometimes accessible on the right, though less often on the left when again pulmonary collapse may distort the normal anatomy, obliging the operator to resort to a fibre optic bronchoscope using the flexible cryoprobes. The first cryoprobes that we used were too short and this was the reason for some technical failures.

Occasionally a flexible probe has ruptured without harm to the patient when they were first being used experimentally : gas leaks occured which resulted in less efficient freezing. Indeed the cryoprobes should always be tested for leaks prior to use. Although the flexible cryoprobes are delicate they rarely cause trouble now.

References

1. Maiwand MO (1987) Cryotherapy for advanced carcinoma of bronchi and trachea. Cryotherapy 9 : 22-24
2. Rayel-Boisdron C (1989) Cryothérapie en pathologie trachéo-bronchique. Thesis. Nancy University, France
3. Homasson JP, Renault P, Angebault M, Bonniot JP, Bell NJ (1986) Bronchoscopic cryotherapy for airway strictures caused by tumors. Chest 90 : 159-164
4. Guichenez P (1989) Expérience de 3 ans de la cryothérapie endobronchique par sonde semi-rigide. A propos de 107 traitements. Thesis, Saint-Étienne University, France
5. Roullier A (1987) Place de la bronchocryothérapie dans le cadre d'une stratégie curatrice des cancers bronchiques. Bull GECC : 1-9
6. Farlet D (1986) Cryothérapie en pneumologie (thesis). Pierre et Marie Curie University, Paris, France

Other endoscopic interventions

Jean-Paul Homasson

The first bronchoscopy was carried out by Killian (Fig. 1) in 1897 to remove a bone from the main bronchus of an old man. Rigid bronchoscopes have been used for diagnostic and therapeutic purposes until around 1970. With the advent of flexible fibreoptic bronchoscopes the equipment had almost been phased out until recently. There is now a resurgence in its use for interventional endoscopic techniques such as cryosurgery, laser therapy or stent insertions. However the fibreoptic bronchoscope is still indicated with the improved equipment being developed such as the fibre optic laser and flexible cryoprobes, even if it is preferable to use a rigid bronchoscope whenever possible. In view of the facility and safety of cryosurgery it is hoped that it will be used sensibly and within the limitations of its capabilities. Finally endobrachytherapy with high dose rates is a new technique available to endoscopists.

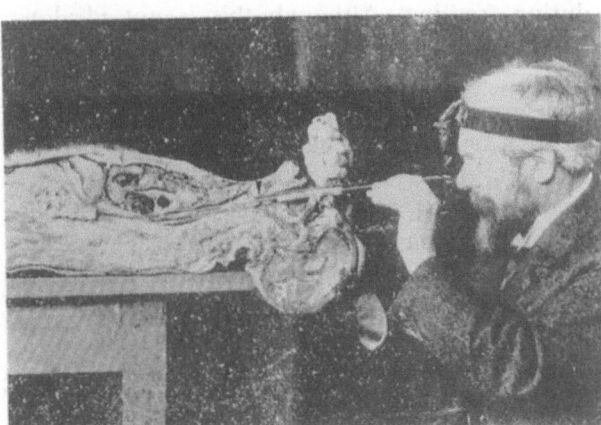

Fig. 1. Killian

All these techniques have their specific indications but they may be combined — for example the combination of laser with cryosurgery will be discussed in the chapter on therapeutic combinations.

Primarily cryosurgery is a method of relieving bronchial obstruction but other more crude techniques have been used since the beginning of bronchoscopy such as forceps dissection. These different techniques will be reviewed and their indications and advantages or contraindications will be highlighted.

Forceps

Bronchial obstructions have been removed with forceps but they are rarely used alone these days as there are more efficient means available. Dissecting forceps carry the risk of serious haemorrhage and although coagulating forceps may diminish this risk it is sometimes difficult to find the optimum level of electrocoagulation. This method, when used in the wrong hands may damage the tracheo-bronchial cartilagenous rings leading to perforation or stricture formation. When compared to cryotherapy Carpenter [1] demonstrated a clearly superior result with cryotherapy. As was discussed in a previous chapter, healing after cryotherapy produced excellent results with a complete restoration of ciliated epithelium and a normal bronchial architecture with no wound retraction or secondary stenosis formation. It should be noted that there is also a risk of secondary haemorrhage with the shedding of slough following electrocoagulation.

Endobronchial electrocautery

The use of endobronchial electrocautery as a tool for use in the management of obstructive endobronchial disease has been reported by Hooper [2], it has both diagnostic and therapeutic applications. The method utilizes two techniques. The first is looping or lassoing of tissue with a wire snare, then resecting the base of the tissue with electrocautery. In the second technique a cautery probe is directly applied to burn, dessicate and vaporize obstructing tissue.

The electrocautery snare can be used to obtain large biopsies of airway lesions, to debulk and remove malignant tissue in the airway, and to treat benign lesions [3]. Application of the endobronchial cautery wire snare requires a configuration of tissue that allows ensnaring a portion of the material for removal. Its most dramatic application is in polypoid abnormalities with small base attachments. With this anatomy, it may be possible to ensnare the complete abnormality and remove it in one piece. Flat lesions or those with large base attachments do not always lend themselves to this type of removal. A snare may only be able to ensnare a small portion of the tissue to be removed and several applications may be necessary for removal of the bulk of the tissue.

In fact this technique is not used extensively and its use should be explored by chest physicians. However there are complications : bleeding and perforation although the potential for perforation and bleeding is probably greater with use of electrocautery probes when used for tissue destruction than it is with a snare.

The equipment is cheap and in combination with cryotherapy would be feasible for removal of lesions with a large base.

Laser

The first tracheal lesions to be treated by lasers were carried out by M.S. Strong in 1974 [4] using a CO_2 laser. In 1977 L. Toty experimented in animals using the YAG Nd laser, then published his first results for its use in humans [5]. Since that time the laser has become without doubt the standard technique for managing bronchial obstructions. The YAG Nd laser is the one most frequently used in interrupted or continuous shots at high energy to vaporize tissue or at low strength (less than 100 Watts, to obtain a photocoagulative effect). Most operators use the fibre optic laser via a rigid bronchoscope under general anaesthetic [6-8]. Some operators have used the laser with a fibre optic bronchoscope and local anaesthesia. This technique does cause problems due to the production of quantities of smoke especially under local anaesthetic.

The complications of laser therapy are well known and occur relatively frequently. They are : perforation of the bronchial wall (the incidence of pneumothorax with laser treatment is around 1 %) ; significant haemorrhage (0.2-10 %) which may be fatal ; hypoxaemia and endobronchial fire [9]. The use of laser therapy requires significant training which is not the case with cryotherapy.

The laser produces immediate relief of bronchial obstruction and this is its main advantage over other modalities. It is therefore the treatment of choice in cases of acute tracheal obstruction leading to respiratory distress, whether caused by tumour or not.

In all other situations where there is no surgery, cryotherapy may be used equally as their indications are identical. In fact cryotherapy has the advantage of being easier to use, with less complications and being considerably cheaper.

The two techniques may be complimentary : cryotherapy may destroy lesions difficult to treat with a laser ; infiltrating lesions and total bronchial stenoses. Using flexible cryoprobes it is even possible to destroy tumours in small bronchi without direct vision which would be unthinkable using a laser. The tumour is located with the fibre optic bronchoscope in place and when the cryoprobe is introduced into the endoscope because of the angle, direct vision is not possible during freezing. Although this is not ideal we have obtained good results with this method without complications.

Regrowth of tumour seems to occur more slowly after cryotherapy than after laser therapy and the long term results seem better with fewer recurrences occurring at later onset. These are only impressions which need long term studies to confirm them. Some French authors [10] using the two techniques have compared the indications of laser and cryotherapy for the same type of lesions (Table 1).

Photochemotherapy using dye laser has not been used frequently and the indications are restricted as photochemotherapy can only destroy small tumours which are equally amenable to cryotherapy. The disadvantages of haematopor-

Table 1. Comparative indications of cryotherapy and laser (after Vergnon, 1987)

Indications	Laser	Cryotherapy
Severe tracheal obstruction	+ + +	No (delayed effect)
Polypoid tumour partial obstruction (trachea — bronchi)	+ + +	+ +
Total bronchial obstruction	Difficult	+ + +
Infiltrating stenosis	No	+ +
Carcinoma *in situ*	No	+ +
Post radiotherapy lesion	Care	+ +
Granuloma	+ + +	+ + +
Haemoptisis from accessible lesions	+	+ + +
Biopsies of haemorrhagic tumours	No	+ + +

phyrine mean that more research should be done to discover other more suitable agents. Laser and cryotherapy may be used together as will be seen in a later chapter.

Brachytherapy

Endobronchial brachytherapy for the treatment of bronchogenic carcinoma was employed in 1921 by Yankauer who treated a patient with repeated applications of encapsulated radium introduced through a rigid bronchoscope [11].

Since then this technique has continued to be used but only in a few countries. Many radiotherapists are opposed to it's use because of the complications, namely perforations and pneumothorax, haemoptysis, tracheo-oesophageal fistulae, movement of the radioactive source, not to mention irradiation of the operator or other team members. The aim is to insert radioactive elements (e.g. Radium 222, Gold 198 or Cobalt 60) directly into the tumours where they are left in place. The problem is that the dose of radiation delivered is not precice. The procedure is carried out using a rigid bronchoscope under general anaesthetic. It is a purely palliative treatment and satisfactory results have been obtained by several authors [12-14]. One improvement was to introduce the source using a fibre optic bronchoscope [15, 16]. The main improvement to the technique is the use of high dose rates which allow irradiation of only a few minutes. The afterloading catheter is introduced via the nose or the mouth and positioned at the site of stenosis under direct vision through a fibreoptic bronchoscope. The procedure is carried out under local anaesthetic and the technique becomes ambulatory.

There are several types of equipment using Iridium 192 [17]. Nevertheless the ultimate development of the research seems to be the micro Selectron HDR, which allows the use of multiple small catheters (Fig. 2) and computerised dosimetry for complete control of the endobronchial radiation dose and field.

The results of authors using this equipment have been gathered [18] and it is the same equipment that we use [19-20].

Brachytherapy is often associated with preliminary laser treatment. We have even used it in conjunction with cryotherapy in a few cases. It is a form of complimentary treatment which produces a good result which may last a long time. One would think that it would have indications as a curative treatment (Fig. 3) but it will always remain a palliative treatment in carcinoma of the bronchus. It is a relatively cheap form of radiotherapy and it may be associated with external irradiation. It is however very expensive compared to laser therapy and even more so compared to cryotherapy.

The indications for HDR brachytherapy have yet to be determined and this technique requires a close collaboration between chest physician and radiotherapist. There are relatively few complications but they remain the same as for other forms of radiotherapy.

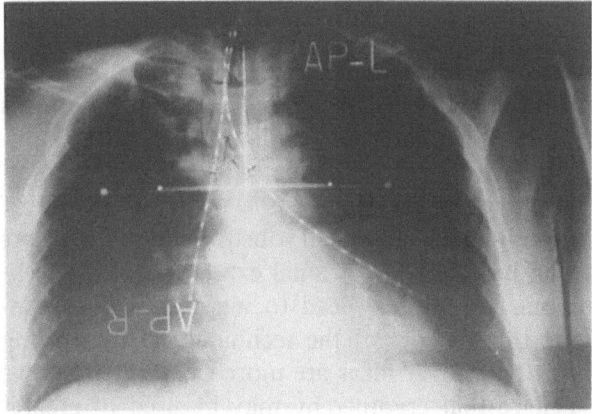

Fig. 2. Radiograph with two catheters (squamous cell carcinoma of the carina)

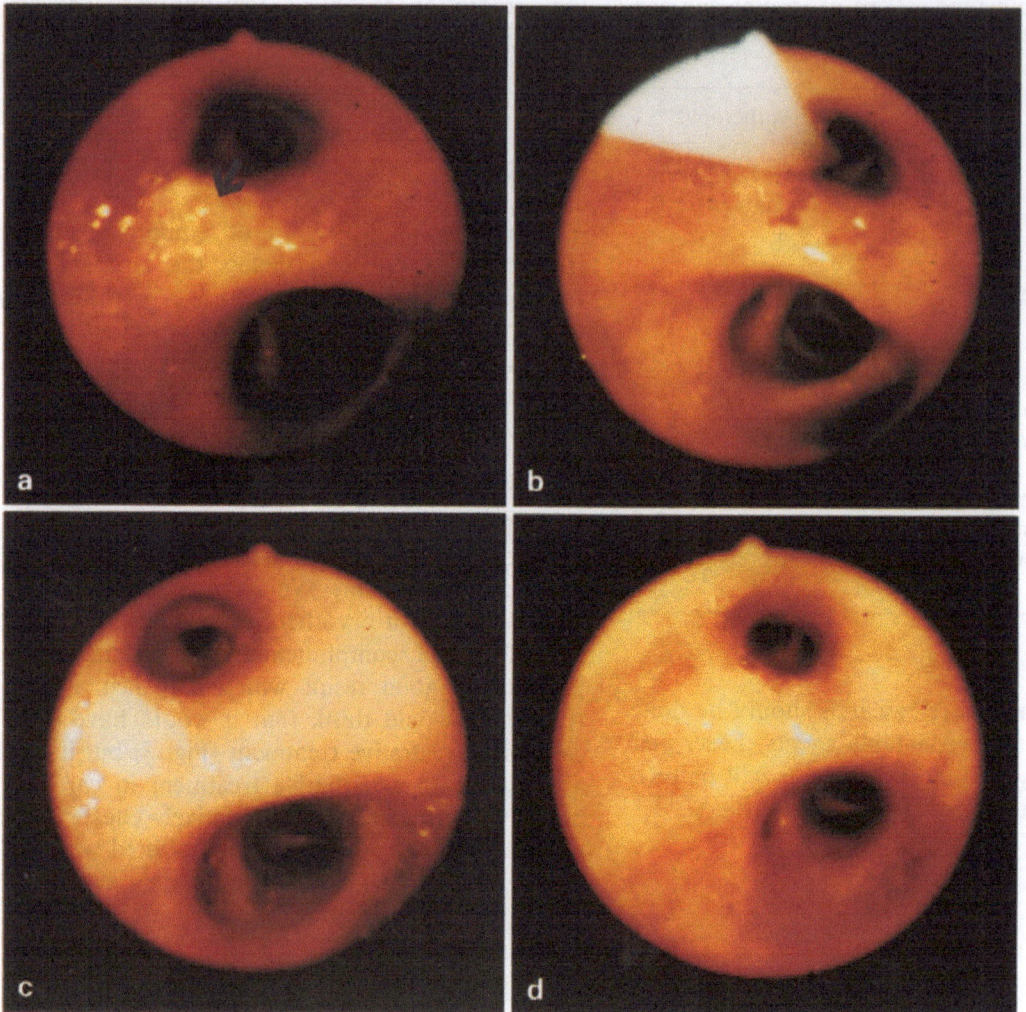

Fig. 3. a Small neoplastic spot on the middle lobe bronchus (recurrence of disease following left pneumonectomy), **b** Catheter introduced into middle lobe, **c** Tumour slough, **d** Result after three months

Conclusion

The chest physician has several techniques at his disposal in his fight against cancer. Rather than the methods competing against each other we think it is preferable to evaluate the indications of each method with a view to using the optimum method alone or in combination. Cryotherapy is often mentioned as a possible method of dealing with bronchial obstruction by authors who have had no personal experience of the technique — this may lead to inaccuracies concerning the benefits of the technique. If by reading this book their ideas are more clearly focused we believe that cryotherapy may be used to greater effect alone or in association with other methods. Cryotherapy, laser, electrocauterization and the insertion of stents all form part of the therapeutic arsenal — each technique having its advantages and disadvantages which should be well understood before the choice is made to treat each individual patient.

References

1. Carpenter RJ, Neel HB, Sanderson DR (1977) Comparison of endoscopic cryosurgery and electrocoagulation of bronchi. Trans Am Acad Ophtalmol Otolaryngol 84 : 313-323
2. Hooper RG, Jackson FM (1985) Endobronchial electrocautery. Chest 87 : 712-714
3. Hooper RG, Jackson FM (1988) Endobronchial electrocautery. Chest 94 : 595-598

4. Strong MS, Vaughan CW, Polnyi T, Wallace R (1974) Bronchoscopic carbon dioxide laser surgery. Ann Otol Rhinol Laryngol 83 : 769-776

5. Toty L (1979) Personne C, Colchen A. Utilisation d'un faisceau laser YAG à conducteur souple, pour le traitement endoscopique de certaines lésions trachéo-bronchiques. Rev Mal Resp 7 : 475-482

6. Dumon JF, Reboud E, Garbe L, Aucomte F, Meric B (1982) Treatment of tracheo-bronchial lesions by laser photoresection. Chest 81 : 278-284

7. Personne C, Colchen A, Leroy M, Vourch G, Toty L (1986) Indications and technique for endoscopic laser resections in bronchology. A critical analysis based upon 2284 resections. J Thorac Cardiovasc Surg 91 : 710-715

8. Cavalière S, Foccoli P, Farina PL (1988) Nd YAG laser bronchoscopy. A five year experience with 1396 applications in 1 000 patients. Chest 94 : 15-21

9. Vanderschueren RGJRA, Westermann CJJ (1990). Complications of endobronchial Neodynium-Yag (Nd = Yag) Laser application. Lung 168 (suppl) : 1089-1094

10. Vergnon JM, Boucheron S, Bonamour D, Fournel P, Emonot A (1987) Destruction endobronchique des lésions tumorales : laser ou cryotherapie ? Rev Pneumol Clin 43 : 19-25

11. Yankauer S (1922) Two cases of lung tumour treated bronchoscopically. NY Med J 115 : 741-742

12. Schlungbaum W, Blum H, Brandt HJ (1962) Ergebnisse der endobronchialen Strahlentherapie des bronchuskarzinoms. Radiologia Austriaca 13 : 201-204

13. Hilaris BS, Martini N (1979) Interstitial brachytherapy in cancer of the lung : a 20 year experience. Int J Rad Oncol Biol Phys 5 : 1951-1956

14. Ledingham SJM, Goldstraw P (1989) Diathermy resection and radioactive gold grains for palliation of obstruction due to recurrence of bronchial carcinoma after external irradiation. Thorax 44 : 48-51

15. Moylan D, Strubler KL, Unal A, Mohiuddin M, Giampetro A, Boon R (1983) Work in progress. Transbronchial brachytherapy of recurrent bronchogenic carcinoma : a new approach using the flexible fiberoptic bronchoscope. Radiology 147 : 253-254

16. Rabie T, Wilson RK, Easley JD, Teague RB, Bloom K, Lawrence EC, Ilaria R (1986) Palliation of bronchogenic carcinoma with 198[Au] Implantation using the fiberoptic bronchoscope. Chest 90 : 641-645

17. Macha HN, Koch K, Stadler M, Schumacher W, Krumhaar D (1987) New technique for treating occlusive and stenosing tumours of the trachea and main bronchi. Endobronchial irradiation by high dose iridium 192 combined with laser canalisation. Thorax 42 : 511-515

18. Activity. Selectron brachytherapy journal. Suppl. 1, 1990. Pulmonary brachytherapy. Nucletron — Leersum, the Netherlands

19. Tredaniel J, Homasson JP, Baud D, Roden S, Hennequin C, Sire C, Maylin C, Hirsch A (1990) Curie thérapie endoluminale a haut débit dans les cancers bronchiques. Technique, indications potentielles, résultats préliminaires. Rev Mal Resp 7 (suppl 3) : R 207

20. Homasson JP, Roden S, Angebault M, Baud D, Hennequin C, Chotin G, Maylin C (1992) Traitement des cancers bronchiques par curiethérapie à haut débit de dose. Presse Med 21 : 317

Cryotherapy and other treatments

Jean-Paul Homasson, Alain Pecking and Jean-Michel Vergnon

In the preceding chapter we discussed the various endoscopic techniques available to the chest physician. These techniques are used to treat cancerous lesions in 80 % of cases. Cryotherapy may be associated with other modalities for the treatment of bronchial carcinoma, for example radiotherapy and chemotherapy — these are studies which have been initiated but they are hardly beyond the experimental stage, however early results are encouraging and there seems to be a possible synergistic effect of combined cryotherapy with both radiotherapy and chemotherapy. If a synergistic effect is proven then the indications for cryotherapy will obviously be widened.

Cryotherapy and forceps

Rodgers [1, 2] has used this technique in the treatment of benign subglottic, tracheal and bronchial stenoses in children as outlined in a preceding chapter.

The stenotic area was first frozen and then dissected with biopsy forceps. We have used this method to remove polypoid stenoses to reduce haemorrhage due to the haemostatic effect of ice, however if there is no urgency, we prefer to wait for the cryonecrosis in order to avoid damaging vessels with the forceps.

It also has to be said that most of the patients treated by Rodgers would normally now be treated with laser either alone or in association with cryotherapy.

Cryotherapy and laser

The combination of therapies would appear to be much more beneficical to patients and has been used by several authors [3, 4] who use one of two techniques. If the obstruction is severe and relief must be procured as an emergency, then the laser should be used first to remove the obstruction. Cryotherapy may then be applied to the remainder of the lesion once the risk of asphyxia has passed. In malignant obstructions for example Lamy used laser therapy to remove the obstruction first, but immediately this occurs vision is often reduced due to a surge of purulent discharge or haemorrhage and at this point he uses cryotherapy to treat any lesions distal to the major obstruction. The cryoprobe may also be used to remove particles of the orginal obstruction which may have fallen into distal bronchi. These are removed using the cryoadherence effect of the frozen tip of the probe.

The combination of cryosurgery-laser treatment may particularly be used to treat benign cuff like stenoses of the trachea, even though it is recognized that cryotherapy is not very effective in treating fibrous lesions. The stenosis is first treated with the laser and when the cartilaginous tracheal rings are nearly exposed, instead of stopping the session the final treatment is done with cryotherapy both to remove the burnt particles and also to treat the bed of the lesion. Using this technique a non retractile scar is obtained which is better than that obtained with the laser alone. A recurrence or a restenosis is either avoided or occurs less frequently than when a laser is used alone.

When used in this order the two modalities are complementary. However other authors [5] have used cryotherapy as a haemostatic procedure before laser application, especially when the tumour to be treated is very vascular ; they freeze the tumour and a few minutes later destroy it with the laser. We think that this is not a good method of using cryotherapy and is due in part to a lack of understanding on behalf of the authors of the true indications of the two methods and of the process of cryodestruction, because if the tumour is completely frozen it will be destroyed in any event, and if there is no urgency then there is no need to follow up the destruction using a laser. If the two methods are used in combination it is with the aim of reducing the danger of lasers and this does not apply if used in this order. The methods of Lamy and Vergnon are the two methods in which a combination of modalities should be employed (see Thesis of Guichenez [4]).

Cryotherapy and chemotherapy

A surprisingly favourable outcome of several cases treated with this combination of therapies merits further study. It has been shown in previous studies [6] that chemotherapy has been more effective following cryotherapy such that a synergistic effect is obtained. Anti cancer drugs would appear to accumulate in the tumour site immediately following cryotherapy. Using an experimental murine tumour preparation, Ikekawa [7] investigated the efficacy of cryochemotherapy and confirmed the phenomenon of trapping of anti-cancer drugs after combined treatment.

We have carried out a preliminary study on 12 patients, the aim of this study was to confirm these experimental findings. The patients who all had inoperable bronchial carcinoma with endobronchial tumour obstructing one main bronchus were treated with bleomycin labelled with cobalt 57 before and after cryotherapy.

The endoscopic treatment was carried out as described before [8] using either a rigid cryoprobe passed through a rigid bronchoscope or else a flexible cryoprobe passed down a fibre optic bronchoscope. The tumour was frozen under direct vision.

Bleomycin (BLM) labelled with Co57 was used as an imaging medium for the assessment of tumour uptake after cryotherapy. The labelling

was carried out using a simple contact of a solution of 15 mg of BLM (Roger-Bellon Laboratories) diluted in 4.5 ml of isotonic saline with 0.65 ml of 0.5 N hydrochloric acid solution of carrier free cobalt 57 chloride at room temperature. The final pH of the solution was adjusted to 4.5 using sodium hydroxide. This radio labelled BLM has been established as being a reliable tumour detector.

The tumour uptake of the radiolabelled BLM has been studied by Rasher [9] and by Taylor [10]. The maximum amount of radioactivity was found either in the mitochondrial fractions for Co57 BLM or lysosomes and cytoplasm with 111 In BLM. These discrepancies related to the radionuclide used suggesting that BLM might only serve as a vector for the radioactive metal. Nevertheless the tumour to blood ratio as well as the tumour to normal ratio were high enough to enable positive tumour detections. Based on this data we carried out a phase one trial on patients with bronchogenic carcinoma where cryotherapy was indicated as a palliative therapy. 15 mg of radiolabelled BLM was injected intravenously. The patient was placed under a gammacamera aimed at the chest. Detection was carried out for 40 minutes on a Sopha imaging computer in frame mode (3 frames/min). A region of interest (ROI) was drawn over the left ventricule in order to plot a time activity curve corresponding to the disappearance of the radiolabelled BLM from the blood. First and second half-lives of the radiolabelled BLM were calculated from this curve and from additional later points obtained from static images performed 1, 2, 3, 4 and 24 hours after injection. For the first two patients delayed images were performed after 48, 72 and 96 hours. As the maximum tumour uptake was obtained between 4 and 24 hours delayed images were abandoned in subsequent cases. Two identical ROI's were drawn on the 4 and 24 hours images. The first ROI was located over tumour and the second ROI over normal tissue. A tumour to normal tissue ratio was then calculated. As the washout time of radiolabelled BLM was about 10 days, the same protocol was performed 15 days later 1 hour after cryotherapy.

All parameters, plasma half-lives and clearance of the radiolabelled BLM tumour/normal tissue ratio obtained before and after cryotherapy were compared using a Student's t test and a Wilcoxon test for correlations.

The tumour to normal tissue ratio evolution according to time was followed on the first two patients. The maximum value was obtained between 4 and 24 hours with a plateau for the delayed values. All tumour to normal tissue ratios were subsequently calculated on the 4 hours images. The results are summarized in Table 1. A significant difference was found regarding tumour uptake of radiolabelled BLM before and after cryotherapy (Fig. 1). The pharmacokinetic data are summarized in Table II.

Most of the cases [1, 2, 4, 5, 7-12] showed an improvement in the kinetic parameters of second half-life and plasma clearance — in two cases [3, 6] we did not see any significant difference before and after treatment. A direct correlation has been demonstrated between the tissue distribution of radiolabelled BLM and the second half-life. The comparison of second half-life mean values obtained before and after cryotherapy demonstrated a significant difference ($p = 0.01$) with a faster second half-life after cryotherapy.

The principles of cryodestruction have been discussed in a previous chapter and as we explained there is an immediate physical effect of both intra and extracellular crystallization [11] followed by a vascular effect [12-13] the vessels are initially constricted — this is followed by vasodilation and hyperaemia followed by stasis. Modification of the vascular endothelium occurs with an increase in the permeability of the vessel walls and increased blood viscosity. Thrombosis and complete circulatory arrest develop as a consequence. The result is a slough which occurs several days later. At the edge of the frozen area the hypothermia causes a heterogenous destructive effect and it is

Table 1. Comparison of the tumour to tissue ratio obtained before and after cryotherapy

Tumour/tissue ratio

	Before	After	Difference %
1	3.422	3.935	15.0
2	2.581	2.930	13.5
3	1.131	1.187	05.0
4	1.652	2.015	22.0
5	2.145	2.784	29.8
6	1.536	3.233	110.5
7	1.652	2.254	36.4
8	2.075	2.926	41.0
9	1.806	1.975	09.4
10	2.101	2.685	27.8
11	2.075	2.926	41.0
12	1.806	1.975	09.4
m sd	1.998 ± 0.579	2.568 ± 0.724	30.00 ± 28.29
t p	2.129 0.04	ddl 22	

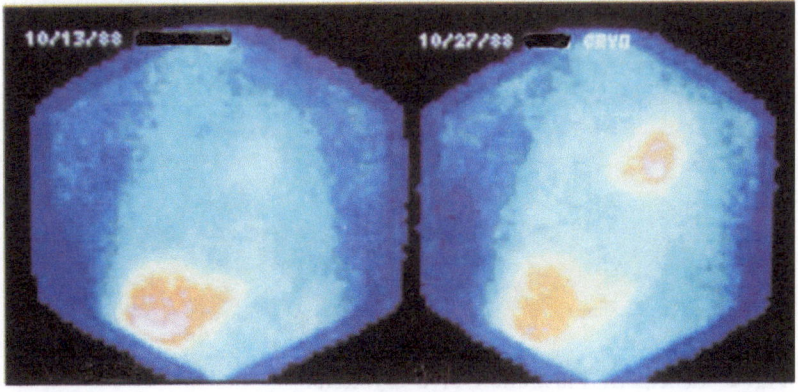

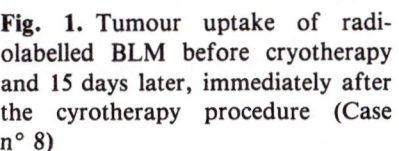

Fig. 1. Tumour uptake of radiolabelled BLM before cryotherapy and 15 days later, immediately after the cyrotherapy procedure (Case n° 8)

Table 2. Pharmacokinetic results obtained from the time-activity curve plotted from the external detection

	First half-life (minutes)		Second half-life (minutes)		Clearance (mg/min)	
	Prior	After	Prior	After	Prior	After
1	1.452	0.545	80.21	14.57	0.105	0.896
2	0.471	0.731	52.92	27.77	0.180	0.349
3	1.131	0.734	34.74	27.52	0.236	0.228
4	0.883	1.435	40.45	32.37	0.198	0.231
5	1.824	1.813	29.39	21.45	0.192	0.283
6	0.754	0.891	21.15	19.45	0.366	0.446
7	1.273	1.964	59.62	49.14	0.192	0.219
8	1.685	0.361	38.74	26.39	0.247	0.851
9	1.551	0.862	122.09	88.63	0.062	0.126
10	1.490	1.288	79.12	60.87	0.106	0.154
11	1.163	0.589	29.81	19.38	0.327	0.779
12	0.466	0.443	16.99	11.61	0.715	0.947
mean	1.179	0.971	50.43	34.10	0.244	0.459
sd	± 0.454	±0.533	± 30.53	± 22.38	±0.172	± 0.315
t	1.201		3.073		− 2.866	
p	NS		0.010		0.015	

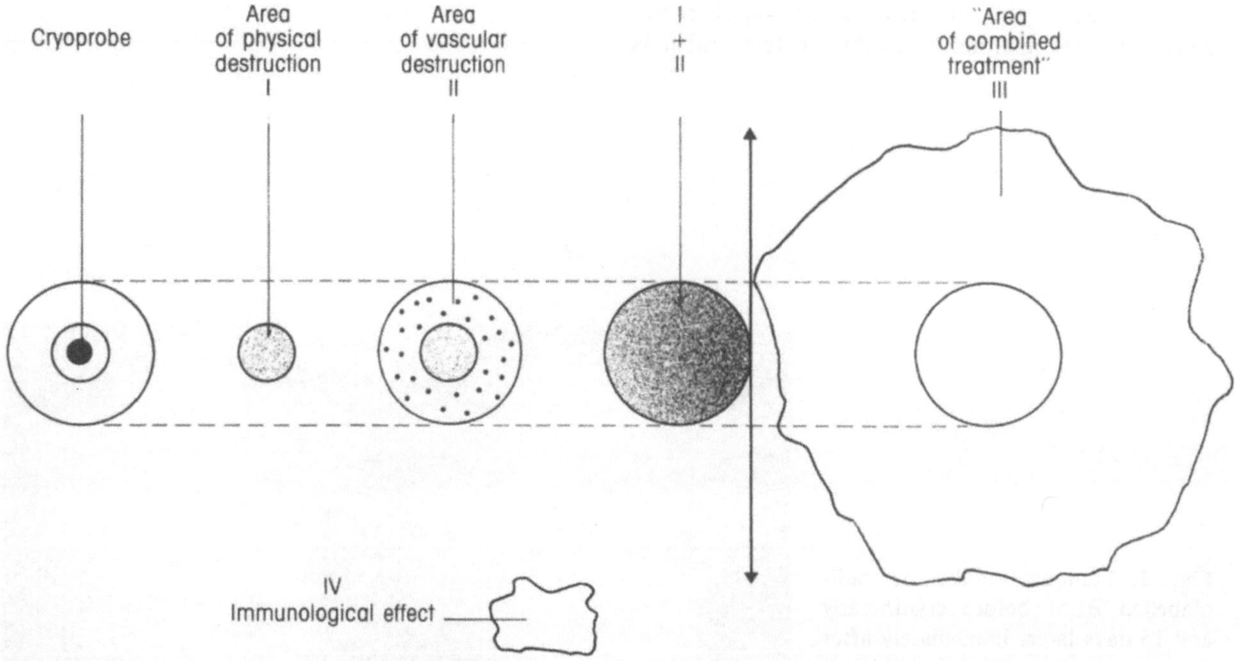

Fig. 2. Schematic illustration of a cryolesion

in these areas that the chemotherapy (or radiotherapy) has a complimentary destructive effect. This is the reason that we have called this area the combined therapeutic area (Fig. 2). This mechanism of the cryodestructive process offers an explanation of the combined therapeutic effects with chemotherapy due to trapping of the anti cancer drugs in the damaged tumour and immediately surrounding areas.

Many studies have demonstrated the affinity of BLM for cancerous bronchial tissue [13] and the value of Cobalt labelled BLM for the detection of these tumours. Nieweg [14] in a study of 268 patients showed a sensibility of 95 % and a specificity of 87 % with a good correlation between the level of fixation and the size of tumour. Thus Cobalt labelled BLM seemed the logical choice as a marker before and after cryotherapy.

The effectiveness of an anti-cancer drug is directly linked to its tissue concentration. In this study we have been able to demonstrate an increase in the uptake of cobalt labelled BLM when the drug is administered intravenously between 2-6 hours following cryotherapy. This represents the time of maximal trapping of BLM at the tumour site and the increase is of the order of 30 % following cryotherapy. There is a significant difference in BLM fixing before and after cryotherapy and the concentration is higher in the frozen zone compared to the untreated zone.

The pharmacokinetic parameters demonstrate that after cryotherapy only the second half life is statistically modified which is in favour of a greater passage into the tissues. This is confirmed by the accelerated plasma clearance.

There is a direct positive correlation between the ratio of tumour/healthy tissue uptake and the increased plasma clearance of BLM. Thus one can postulate that the BLM is trapped in the tumour zone as a consequence of the vascular disruption caused by freezing.

Our study thus confirms the experimental findings of Ikekawa in the mouse and offers an explanation for the initial clinical findings reported by Benson [6] in ENT tumours treated with chemotherapy in association with cryotherapy. Our initial clinical results seem to confirm that chemotherapy may be more effective after cryotherapy : tumor destruction is superior to that found with chemotherapy alone and that survival time has exceeded two years in some patients who were inoperable at the outset. The histology of the tumour did not influence the nuclear measurements. At present the series is too small and the

results too few to draw any meaningful conclusions.

When surgical resection is unfeasible, cryochemotherapy could be a regimen for the treatment of bronchial carcinomas. Nevertheless large scale controlled trials need to be carried out to test the efficacy of such combined forms of therapy.

References

1. Rodgers BM, Talbert JL (1978) Clinical application of endotracheal cryotherapy. J Ped Surg 13 : 662-668
2. Rodgers BM, Moazam F, Talbert JL (1983) Endotracheal cryotherapy in the treatment of refractory airway strictures. Ann Thor Surg 35 : 52-57
3. Rayel-Boisdron C (1989) La cryothérapie en pathologie trachéo-bronchique (Thesis) Nancy University, France
4. Guichenez P (1989) Expérience de 3 ans de la cryothérapie endobronchique par sonde semi-rigide. A propos de 107 traitements (Thesis). Saint-Etienne University, France
5. Personne C, Colchen A, Bonnette P, Leroy M, Bisson A (1990) Laser in bronchology : Methods of application. Lung (suppl) 168 : 1085-1088
6. Benson JW (1975) Combined chemotherapy and cryosurgery for oral cancer. Am J Surg 13 : 596-600
7. Ikekawa S, Ishihara K, Tanaka S, Ikeda S (1985) Basic studies of cryochemotherapy in a murine tumor system. Cryobiology 22 : 477-483
8. Homasson JP, Renault P, Angebault M, Bonniot JP, Bell NJ (1986) Bronchoscopic cryotherapy for airway strictures caused by tumors. Chest 90 : 153-184
9. Rasker JJ (1975) Tumor detection with radioactive isotope labelled bleomycin. Drukkery van der Deren B.V., Groningen
10. Taylor DM, Cottrall MT (1974) Comparison of 57 Co, 69 Zn and 111 In bleomycin complexes for tumour localization. Proc of the International Symposium of Radiopharmaceuticals. Atlanta, USA
11. Gage AA (1969) Cryosurgery for oral and pharyngeal carcinoma. Am J Surg 118 : 669-872
12. Rubinsky B, Pegg DI (1988) A mathematical model for the freezing process in biological tissue. Proc R Soc London 234 : 343-358
13. Svanberg LE (1976) Bleomycin and lung cancer. In : GANN Monograph. 19 on cancer research, 193-220
14. Nieweg OE, Beekhuis H, Piers DA, Slutter HJ, Van Der Wal AM, Woldring MG (1984) Scintigraphy with 57 Co Bleomycin in the detection of lung cancer : a review of 268 well documented patients. Cancer 53 : 1675-1681

Cryotherapy — Radiotherapy

Jean-Michel Vergnon and Jean-Paul Homasson

Selective cellular necrosis represents the main characteristic of tissue destruction brought about by freezing. Two factors contribute to cell death :

• A physical effect with cellular dehydration and extracellular followed by intracellular crystallization [1].

• A vascular effect of microthrombosis [2].

Since 1984, bronchial cryotherapy has been increasingly utilized in France. In endobronchial obstructive lesions, it gives good results in more than 70 % of cases [3-5].

In localised inoperable bronchial carcinomas, radiotherapy is the accepted treatment. The mean survival of patients treated in this way is only 10 months [6] and local eradication of tumour is only obtained in approximately 35 % of cases [7, 8].

In obstructive tumours the regression of atelectasis is achieved after irradiation in only 21 % of cases without local treatments of the disease [9].

Treatment of these obstructive tumours with the YAG laser has been suggested prior to irradiation [10]. This protocol gives better survival and quality of life. Non-resection endoscopically is associated with a poor prognosis [10, 11].

Like laser therapy, cryotherapy will relieve bronchial obstructions and prevent local complications which are the cause of the majority of deaths [12].

Moreover, certain studies have suggested a possible potentialization between cryotherapy and irradiation : in a study of a cryo-lesion of a rabbit oesophagus studied under microangiography, Le Pivert [13] demonstrated the appearance of marked neovascularization of a scar 15 days after cryotherapy. A similar neovascularization has been found after cryotherapy of experimental tumours in rats (Le Pivert, personal communication). This hypervascularization may increase the radio-sensitivity of residual well vascularized cells.

Personal experimental studies

Since 1987 we have studied the production of cyrolesion in a model of small cell bronchial carcinoma grafts in the athymic mouse.

The microscopic appearance of the cryo-lesion 15 days after cryotherapy shows a homogenous destruction of an area of 3 mm surrounding the cryoprobe plus a more peripheral area of piecemeal necrosis sparing parts of the adjacent cells [14]. New vessel formations induced by tumour growth, increase local circulation and thus heat, which slows the progression of freezing thus protecting the cells from the cryo-necrosis (Fig. 1).

The new vessel formation occurring during the healing phase, combined with the intra tumoral necrosis of the less well vascularized area produce a zone which is sensitive to the effects or radiation.

Material and method

Thirty-five patients (32 men, 3 women) who present with obstruction of the trachea or a main or lobar bronchus secondary to inoperable non

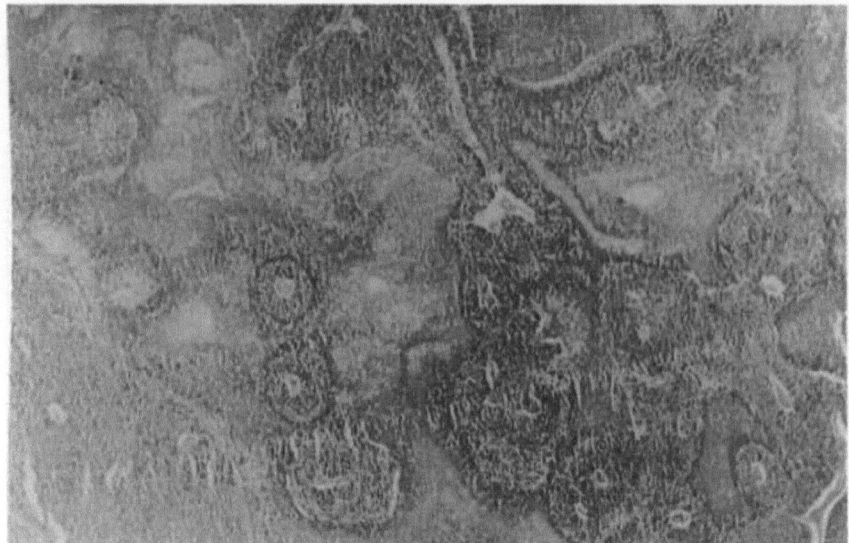

Fig. 1. Light microscope appearance of the peripheral zone of a cryolesion (at 15 days) of a small cell carcinoma of the bronchus grafted onto an athymic mouse. Persistence of islets of viable tumour cells (in violet) surrounding intact vessels. The remainder of the tumour is the site of a homogeneous necrosis (in pink)

small cell bronchial carcinoma and without metastases, were included in our prospective study between March 1986 and March 1990.

These 35 patients were inoperable either due to local reasons (24 cases, group 1). These tumours were classified as stage III b of the classification TNM [15], or due to functional reasons (chronic obstructive airways disease) in the remaining 11 cases (group 2). These tumours werè in stage IIa or IIIa). Thirty-three of the these patients presented with squamous cell carcinoma and 2 with an adenocarcinoma.

The first phase of treatment was cryotherapy under general anaesthesia using a nitrous oxide driven cyoprobe of 3 mm in diameter DATE (France) with an eyepiece bayonet specifically adapted for use via the operative channel (bronchoscope — Vergnon — Wolf, France) (Fig. 2). The cyrotherapy consisted of one session in 19 cases, 2 sessions with an 8 days interval in 13 cases and 3 sessions in 3 cases. A laser resection was required in addition to the first session of cryotherapy in 7 cases because of asphyxiating tracheal stenosis.

The results of cryotherapy were assessed 15 days later by means of fibre optic bronchoscopy. Patients were classified according to a favourable response (more than 50 % tumour destruction at each site of treatment) and an unfavourable response (less than 50 % of tumour destruction). Bronchial biopsy was carried out systematically.

Fifteen to 21 days after cryotherapy curative radiotherapy was commenced : 40 grays in 16 fractions to anterior-posterior fields and 10 days later an additional fraction of 15 grays by tangential field.

The results of radiotherapy were evaluated with fibreoptic bronchoscopy with biopsy one month after the end of irradiation.

The long term follow-up of the patients was carried out without complementary chemotherapy or further cryotherapy, but using local laser or stent treatment when required.

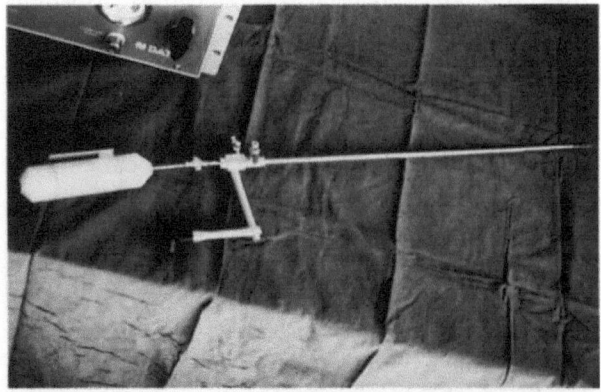

Fig. 2. Cryotherapy equipment. Eye piece with bayonet fixing (Wolf) and semi rigid cryoprobe (DATE) introduced into the operative lumen of a rigid bronchoscope

Results

1) The cryotherapy-radiotherapy was carried out in 33 out of 35 cases, 2 patients received only 35 grays.

The cryotherapy did not produce any significant side-effects. The radiotherapy caused 2 cases of irradiation pneumopathy (1 fatal) and 1 post radiation fibrous tracheal stenosis.

2) Results of cryotherapy (Table 1) — A favourable result was achieved in 23 out of 35 cases with absence of residual detectable lesion.

An unfavourable result occurred in the 12 remaining cases with persistence of tumour histologically confirmed in 10 out of 12 cases.

Results of radiotherapy (Table 1) : after radiotherapy, endoscopic control did not reveal a detectable lesion in 18 of 23 patients (78 %) who showed a favourable response to cryotherapy. In contrast a tumour persisted in cases with an unfavourable response to cryotherapy.

Long-term results — survival

Among the 18 patients followed up, only 8 had local recurrence with 6 of these confirmed histologically (Table 1). The survival curves differ significantly according to the response to cryotherapy (mean 15 months versus 4 months) (Fig. 3). In contrast, surgical contra indication (advanced local disease or functional contraindication) does not modify the survival curves (Figs. 4 and 5).

In the group with a good response to cryother-

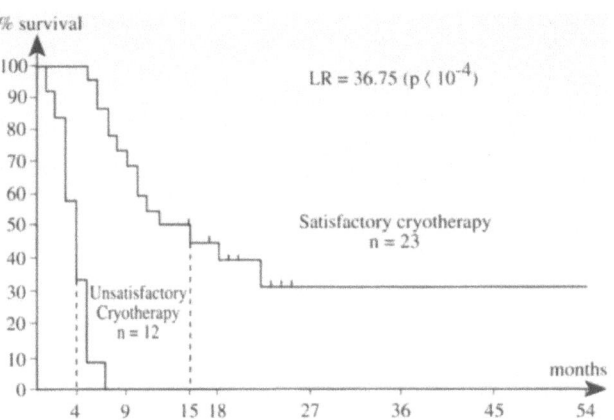

Fig. 3. Survival curves of Kaplan-Meier. Benefit in terms of survival determined by effective cryotherapy. LR : Leg-rank test

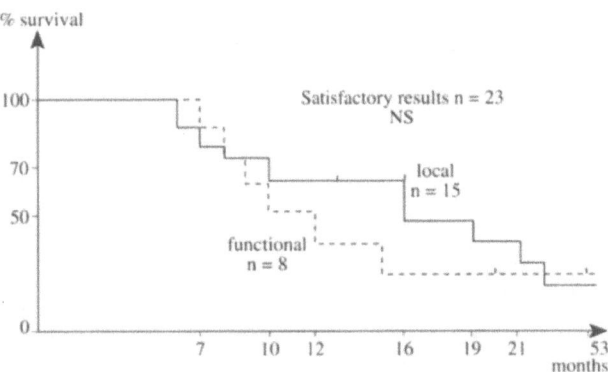

Fig. 4. Effective cryotherapy. Survival according to the reason of surgical contraindication. Absence of significant difference

Table 1. Efficacy of each therapeutic phase assessed on local biopsies : — no eradication of tumour by radiotherapy with ineffective cryotherapy, — eradication of 78 % under radiotherapy in case of effective cryotherapy

	Age years	Group	Negative biopsy after cryotherapy	Available histology Negative biopsy after irradiation	Secondary local relapse
Satisfactory cryotherapy n = 23	66 ± 6.9	14 group 1 9 group 2	7/17 (42 %)	17/22 (78 %)	6/14 (42,8 %)
Unsatisfactory cryotherapy n = 12	58.9 ± 12.9	9 group 1 3 group 2	2/12 (17 %)	0/8 (0 %)	

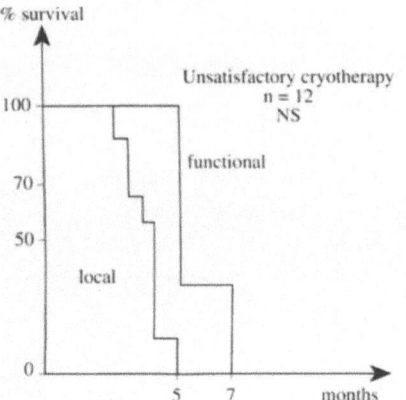

Fig. 5. Ineffective cryotherapy. Survival according to the reason of surgical contraindication. Absence of significant difference

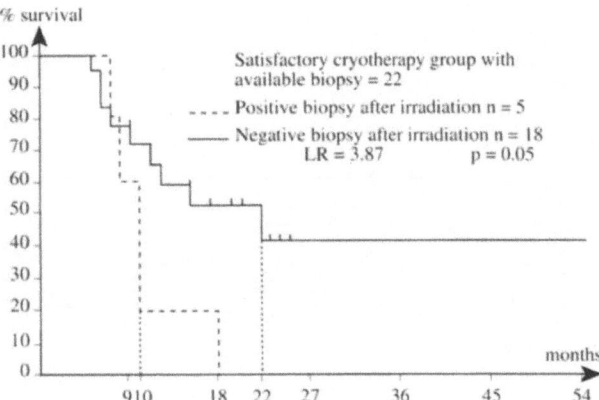

Fig. 6. Effective cryotherapy. Role of effective local control, confirmed histologically of the tumour on survival

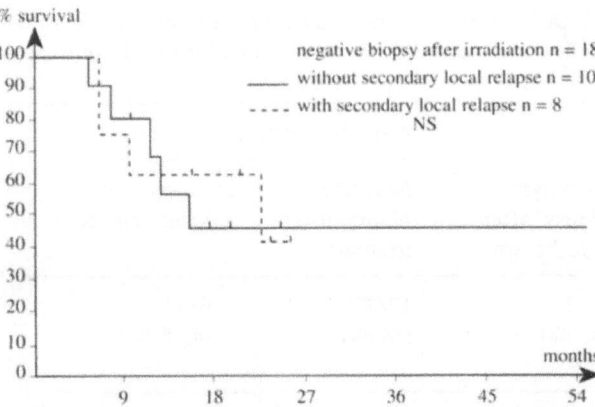

Fig. 7. Effective cryotherapy with local eradication. Absence of influence on survival of an ultimate local relapse. Artwork labels

apy, with histological control of disease, significant improvement of survival was obtained (mean 22 months versus 10 months (Fig. 4). In contrast, the presence or otherwise of a local recurrence did not modify the survival curve (Fig. 5).

Discussion

This non-randomised study does not prove the potentiating effect of cryotherapy on the effect of radiotherapy. However, it confirms several important points.

1) Cryotherapy is a safe method which does not give rise to any premature deaths and is successful in approximately 70 % of cases [4-5].

2) This study reinforces the interest already generated [10-12] of eliminating an obstruction prior to irradiation in order to improve survival and avoid local complications.

The survival curves obtained correspond closely to those obtained with laser [10, 11].

The role of local treatment has especially been underlined in the evolution of local squamous cell cancers [11] which were the preponderant type of cancer in this series.

Furthermore, the presence of local obstruction appears to be an important prognostic criterion, survival being more dependent on this factor than on the TNM stage (same survival whatever the stage).

3) This study also confirms the inadequacy of radiotherapy alone in relieving a bronchial obstruction and achieving local eradication of obstructive tumours [9].

4) The value of local control of tumour after irradiation has already been demonstrated [6]. We confirmed this by showing that survival depends on this eradication even in cases where the mechanical elimination of obstruction is assured (Fig. 4).

We consider that the best survival obtained after cryoradiotherapy partly depends on an initial effective local eradication (78 % against 35 % generally reported in other series) [7, 8]. This « curative » local efficacy raises the possibility of an increased tumour radio-sensitivity, induced by the vascular effects of the cryotherapy. This effect is being looked at experimentally using irradiation alone or after cyrotherapy of bronchial tumours in athymic mice (experiment at present in progress) and by analysis of rate of local eradication of accessible inoperable bronchial neoplams, treated randomly by either cryotherapy and radiotherapy or by radiotherapy alone. This study is being carried out by the cryotherapy group of the French language Pneumology Society.

A similar study carried out by Benis (in collaboration with J.-P. Homasson) in 29 patients gave identical results in inoperable non small cell carcinomas of the bronchus [16].

Association of cryotherapy and high dose rate endobrachytherapy

In the preceding chapter we discussed HDR brachytherapy as a new method of treatment for bronchial carcinoma. Curative indications are rare and it is therefore a palliative method which may be used alone or in association with other therapeutic modalities. Our own study, which at present is the only one, deals in such small numbers that no real conclusion can be drawn on the efficacy or duration of survival when cryotherapy is associated with brachytherapy.

As for the association of external radiotherapy with cryotherapy we have started first with cryotherapy. This step is logical if one considers the possibility of a synergistic effect of the two modalities. The use of cryotherapy initially creates a reduction in tumour volume, if the bronchial obstruction is complete, reopening following cryotherapy allows the passage of catheters throughout the length of the tumour prior to brachytherapy. The indications are thus the same as for laser-brachytherapy [17]. Because of the high cost of brachytherapy it is necessary to specify the indications for its use. They must be different to those of cryotherapy or laser therapy, however the association of cryotherapy-brachytherapy deserves further study as our preliminary results are encouraging. The deep action of brachytherapy completes the local action of freezing and the disappearance of the tumour seems more rapid. Also the use of brachytherapy does not exclude the concurrent use of external irradiation.

References

1. Mazur P (1977) The role of intracellular freezing in the death of cells cooled at supraoptimal rates. Cryobiology 14 : 251-272

2. Gill W, Long WB (1971) A critical look at cryosurgery. Cryosurgery 56 : 344-351

3. Homasson JP, Renault P, Angebault M, Bonniot JP, Bell NJ (1986) Bronchoscopic cryotherapy for airway strictures caused by tumors. Chest 90 : 159-164

4. Homasson JP, Angebault M, Bonniot JP, Baud D, Roden S, François-Coudray S (1990) Cryotherapy of benign and malignant tracheo bronchial tumors. Report of 250 cases (abstract). Chest 98 (suppl) 2 : 131 S

5. Vergnon JM, Guichenez Ph, Fournel P, Emonot A (1990) Efficacy of cryotherapy in bronchial tumors (abstract). Am Rev Resp Dis 141 : 402

6. Petrovich Z, Stanley K, Cox JD, Paig C (1981) — Radiotherapy in the management of locally advanced lung cancer of all cell types. Cancer 48 : 1335-1340

7. Perez CA, Stanley K, Grundy G, Hanson W, Rubin P, Kramer S (1982) — Impact of irradiation technique and tumour extent in tumor control and survival of patients with unresectable non-oat cell carcinoma of the lung report by the radiation therapy oncology group. Cancer 50 : 1091-1099

8. Kjaer M (1982) Radiotherapy of squamous adeno and large cell carcinoma of the lung. Cancer Treat Rev 9 : 1-20

9. Chetty KG, Moran EM, Sassoon CSH, Viravathana T, Light RW (1989). Effects of radiation therapy on bronchial obstruction due to bronchogenic carcinoma. Chest 95 : 582-584

10. Eichenhorn MS, Kvale PA, Miks VM, Seydel HG, Horowitz B, Radke JR (1986) Initial combination therapy with YAG laser photoresection and irradiation for inoperable non small cell carcinoma of the lung. A preliminary report. Chest 89 : 782-785

11. Ross DJ, Mohsenifar Z, Koerner SK (1990). Survival characteristics after neodymium YAG laser photoresection in advanced stage lung cancer. Chest 98 : 581-585

12. Desai SJ, Mehta Ac, Medendorp SV, Golish JA, Ahmad M (1988) — Survival experience following Nd : YAG laser photoresection for primary bronchogenic carcinoma. Chest 94 : 939-944

13. Le Pivert PJ (1980) Basic considerations of the cryolesion. In : Richard J. Ablin (Ed) Handbook of Cryosurgery. Marcel Dekker Inc., New York and Basel, pp. 15-68

14. Vergnon JM, Baril A, Court Fortune I, Boyer Y, Emonot A (1989) — Efficacité et hétérogénéité de la destruction cryothérapique. Étude sur cancer bronchique à petites cellules greffé sur souris NU/NU (Abstract). Rev Mal Resp 6 : 160

15. Mountain CF (1986) — A new international staging system for lung cancer. Chest 89 (suppl 2) 259-339

16. Benis M (1991) Association cryothérapie-radiothérapie dans le traitement des cancers bronc-

hiques non à petites cellules inopérables. Étude de
29 cas. Université René Descartes, Paris V
17. Homasson JP, Roden S, Angebault M, Baud D,

Hennequin C, Chotin G, Maylin C (1992) Traitement des cancers bronchiques par curiethérapie à
haut débit de dose. Presse Med 21 : 317

Cryotherapy of carcinoma in situ and microinvasive carcinomas

Gervais Ozenne

Histopathology

Carcinoma in situ and microinvasive tracheobronchial carcinomas are well defined histological entities. They are characterized by histological changes of the respiratory mucosa which is generally considered to be the site of origin of bronchial cancer, namely malpighian metaplasia, with varying degrees of cellular changes giving the appearance of dysplasia. The criteria which distinguish a carcinoma in situ from dysplasia have been proposed by Black and Akermann [1]. They include the loss of normal cellular differentiation, absence of ciliated and mucous cells, disruption of epithelial architecture and cytonuclear and mitotic abnormalities throughout the entire thickness of the abnormal epithelium. Carcinoma in situ is generally associated with an increase in the thickness of the epithelium, very often with hyperacanthosis [2]. As a rule the borderline between the lesion and normal or dysplastic epithelium is well defined. The adjoining glands and excretory tubes may be invaded with malignant cells whilst preserving the basal membrane.

Microinvasive carcinoma is defined by the penetration of this basal membrane with an infiltration of the mucosal chorion which does not affect the muscular layer [3]. The difference between a carcinoma in situ and a microinvasive carcinoma is at times difficult to establish, the invasive carcinomas may conserve the basal material at the periphery of the infiltrated tubes. The inflammation of a mucosa with exocytosis of inflammatory cells in the surface epithelium alters the basal membrane. This reaction, when occuring in an epithelium with all the characteristics of a carcinoma in situ may raise the suspicion of microinvasive carcinoma. An intact basal membrane is not necessarily an absolute criteria in discriminating between in situ and microinvasive carcinoma : it is also necessary to consider the degree of epithelial and cellular reactions.

The abnormalities of the bronchial mucosa which correspond to this definition are frequently encountered in specimens examined systematically from autopsy or pulmonary excision. Black and Akerman found carcinomas in situ in 33 % of 60 squamous cell bronchial carcinomas, generally in the region of the invasive tumour but also at a distant site in the tracheobronchial tree [1]. Auerbach [2] found them in smokers with a frequency which correlated with the amount of tobacco consumed and even more often in 83 % of subjects who died of bronchial cancer.

There is no longer any doubt that microinvasive carcinomas correspond to the true aggressive carcinoma. This is not necessarily the case with respect to carcinomas in situ which may persist in this non invasive state for an indefinite period without ever transforming into an invasive lesion during the entire life of the patient, they may even regress [4]. There is no morphological criterion to enable us to distinguish between a lesion which will remain quiescent and one with malignant potential.

Clinical observations

In clinical practice distinguishing between carcinoma in situ and microinvasive carcinomas is rarely a problem, in spite of the frequency with which it is found in autopsy specimens.

It appears in a variety of circumstances. A mucosal appearance of this nature can be observed in the bronchial specimens obtained after conventional pulmonary excision for bronchial cancer. This is probably the most frequent case [5]. It presents specific problems which are described in this chapter. Nevertheless, in this instance the fact of having a precise and efficacious technique for local control may complicate the therapeutic problems.

There is currently no specific experience of cryotherapy in respect of the neoplastic recurrences at the sites of pneumonectomy or lobectomy. We will not elaborate further on this aspect of the problem.

Apart from this particular circumstance, the diagnosis of a carcinoma in situ or microinvasive carcinoma may be conducted schematically according to 2 different methods, a purely histological method and an optical method, and in 2 different situations.

When tumour cells are discovered in the bronchial secretions of subjects with normal chest X-rays bronchial endoscopy is carried out, but no lesion is seen under white light examination. The carcinoma in situ or microinvasive carcinomas may then be detected by systematic biopsies taken at random from an inflammatory bronchial mucosa or in biopsies taken after pretreatment with haematoporphyrine [6] or fluorescein [7]. Occasionally, the tumour is only discovered by a histopathological examination of specimens from a pulmonary excision, lobectomy or segmentectomy after localization by means of selective cytological brushings or lavage [8].

The carcinoma may be visible at endoscopy and the appearance of the mucosa indicates the appropriate site for biopsies. The tumour is visible, its limits are well defined, and it has the appearance of a small area of mucosa often rounded and raised and distinguished by its pink or pale colour.

The appearance corresponds to the 'tumourlets' [9] which are more extensive with a rough and slightly wrinkled surface.

It is not certain that the lesions discovered with either of these two methods have the same prognostic significance, even if the histology of the biopsies are similar. The fact that the lesion is visible at endoscopy may indicate a transformation to an aggressive tumour.

Therapy

Surgery

The therapeutic options regarding carcinoma in situ and microinvasive carcinomas depend on the clinical and histopathological findings. Whenever possible conventional pulmonary excision is the treatment of choice in all microinvasive carcinomas and in doubtful carcinoma in situ where a distal lesion is not actually viable. It is also the treatment advocated by most authors in the case of carcinoma in situ confirmed by biopsy. However excision can sometimes make the treatment of another invasive tumour difficult or impossible.

The surgical option is based on several considerations, the impossibility of demonstrating with certainty the in situ character of the lesion (biopsies only represent sample specimens), and the absence of data concerning the long-term results of tumours treated locally (with the disadvantage of local therapy not providing any information regarding lymph node involvement). If local treatment of carcinoma in situ proved to be efficacious in the long-term it would become the treatment of choice. It is less traumatic and of less immediate risk to the patient, also loss of a pulmonary lobe or a lung may make further surgical intervention impossible in cases of recurrence.

Moreover, surgical excision is often impossible because of the underlying poor respiratory function associated with chronic lung disease, the position of the lesion or previous surgery. Local treatment of the tumour is the only possibility in such cases, as chemotherapy is not a treatment option for first time treatment of tracheobronchial carcinoma at present.

Local treatment

Local treatment of carcinoma in situ and microinvasive carcinomas may be undertaken by various methods : external and interstitial radiotherapy and various endoscopic methods : e.g. Laser, dynamic phototherapy, electrocoagulation, cryotherapy, or even by excision biopsy.

Radiotherapy has the advantage of being able to combine local treatment with that of any possible nodular involvement. However, to be effective, high dosage administration of up to 45 Gray is required which prevents subsequent use of this form of therapy in case of recurrence. It has never been advocated or even tested for this indication.

Endoscopic methods for the treatment of superficial carcinomas are still in the experimental stage. To our knowledge there are no series published on the long-term results of carcinoma in situ or microinvasive carcinomas treated with these methods and certainly none comparing them with surgery.

The CO_2 laser has the advantage of precision and control of depth of action which are suitable for superficial lesions, but it is difficult to operate and is limited to areas of the mucosa which can be reached with a rigid bronchoscope. The Nd-YAG laser may be used with a fibreoptic bronchoscope thus permitting treatment of otherwise inaccessible lesions.

Dynamic phototherapy may be used in addition to the diagnostic method of fluorescence of the derivatives of haematoporphyrine accumulated in malignant cells.

Red light induces a photodynamic reaction which produces free radicals of oxygen, these are lethal for the cell which dies within a few days [12]. The red light penetrates to a depth of 2 to 10 mm into the tissues and this method is potentially curative, but it is made less attractive owing to its technical complexity. Some long term controlled cases have been reported [13, 14]. The advantage of dynamic phototherapy is its association with a diagnostic technique, which enables detection of lesions otherwise invisible to examination with white light, and the subsequent precise treatment of such lesions.

Electrocauterization at present is only used occasionally and would appear to be a method worth testing for this indication [15].

Finally, for the very small, endoscopically visible tumours it is possible to obtain complete excision of lesions using biopsy forceps — particularly when using a rigid bronchoscope [16].

Because of its properties, cryotherapy by means of N_2O driven cryoprobes constitutes an effective means of destruction of superficial neoplastic lesions. It has the advantage of being safe to use and easy to manipulate ; of having a complementary haemostatic action and enabling biopsies to be taken immediately after treatment, as well as allowing treatment of more distal, less accessible areas of the tracheobronchial tree.

Despite its novelty, there is already fairly extensive experience of it's use for this indication [17].

Cryotherapy

In 1988 a register of carcinoma in situ and microinvasive carcinomas of the trachea or bronchi treated by cryotherapy was started at the GECC (Groupe d'étude de la cryochirurgie, 8, rue Ambroise-Croizat, 03100 Montluçon, France) in order to monitor the efficacity and limits of this particular indication.

Material and results

By October 1990, 20 tumour sites had been recorded. They satisfied the following criteria : Abnormal tracheobronchial mucosa with clearly defined limits on direct vision, negative radiography and multiple biopsy specimens showing superficial carcinoma in the epithelial or chorion layer without extension into the muscle layer. Several patients were treated simultaneously or successively at several tumour sites : 2 sites for 3 patients and 3 sites for 1 patient. 15 patients were also treated in 6 respiratory medicine units (Table 1).

Table 1. Origin of patients and number of tumours treated by cryotherapy

	Patient origin	
	Patients	Tumours treated with cryotherapy
Rouen	4	7
St-Etienne	5	6
Grenoble	2	3
Tours	2	2
Bordeaux	1	1
Nîmes	1	1
	15	20

Rouen : G. Ozenne ; St-Étienne : J-M. Vergnon ; Grenoble : F. Blanc-Jouvan ; Tours : A. Roullier ; Bordeaux : G. Courty ; Nîmes : M. Taulelle.

In 6 patients the carcinoma in situ was discovered at follow-up after treatment of bronchial carcinoma (4 cases) or ENT malignancy (2 cases). In 9 patients the tumour was a primary neoplastic lesion of the lung.

The distribution of lesions is shown in Figure 1. The sites of the lesions are equally divided between the right and left bronchus : 9 sites in each together with one tracheal tumour and one tumour at the carina.

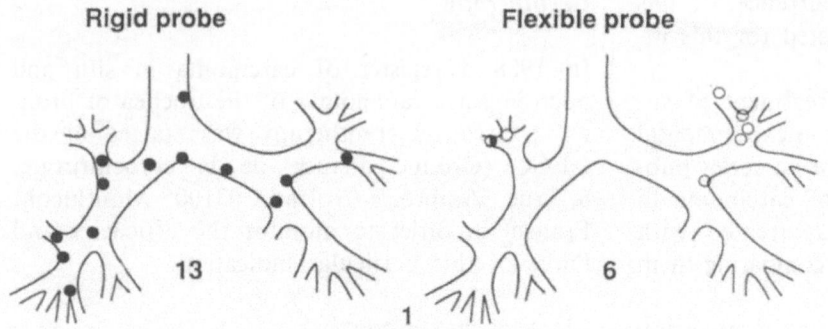

Fig. 1. Distribution of the 13 tumours treated with rigid cryoprobe (black circles left figure) ; 6 tumours treated by flexible cryoprobe (white circles right figure)

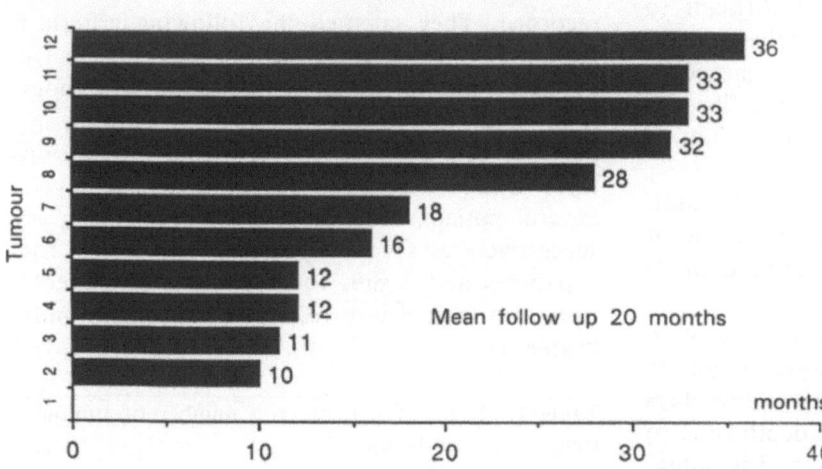

Fig. 2. Endoscopic follow-up of 12 tumours treated by cryotherapy initially without surgery and without recurrence. 20 months follow-up.

Cryotherapy (Fig. 1) : Tumours accessible by rigid bronchoscopy were treated with a rigid probe, apart from a lesion situated at the left interlobar branch. A lesion on the ventral aspect of the right upper lobe bronchus was treated with a flexible probe after an incomplete result with the rigid probe. For 15 tumours cryotherapy was carried out in a single session, for the 5 other tumours, the initial cryotherapy was divided into 2 or more sessions with 1-2 weeks intervals : 3 sessions twice and 6 sessions once.

Initial results : At follow-up bronchoscopy all tumours had disappeared in 19 out of 20 cases. Cytology was negative and biopsies revealed normal or either metaplastic or dysplastic changes only. In some cases this result was delayed for 2 weeks. In one case, situated distally in an apical segment, cryotherapy was ineffective and rapid tumour growth, visible on radiography, required a lobectomy for carcinoma of stage $T_1 N_0$.

Medium term results

Medium term implies the current state of the 19 tumour sites successfully treated.

Thirteen of the 19 patients at present have no endoscopic, histological or cytological evidence of recurrence. One patient had a lobectomy although the excised lobe showed no evidence of malignancy at the site of treatment.

The 12 other tumour sites treated were followed with regular endoscopy (Fig. 2). The average length of follow up being 20 months with the lon-

Medium-term results

Relapse: 6/19

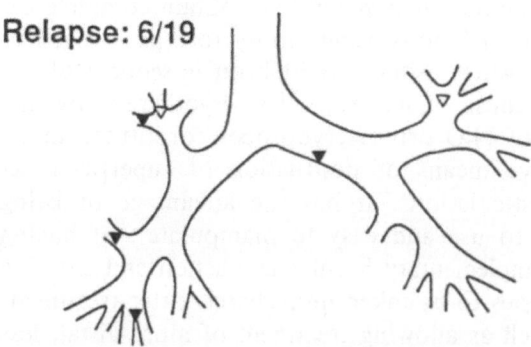

Fig. 3. Distribution of recurrence after initial treatment with cryotherapy alone. Black triangle indicates initial treatment with rigid cryoprobe ; white triangle : indicates initial treatment with flexible cryoprobe

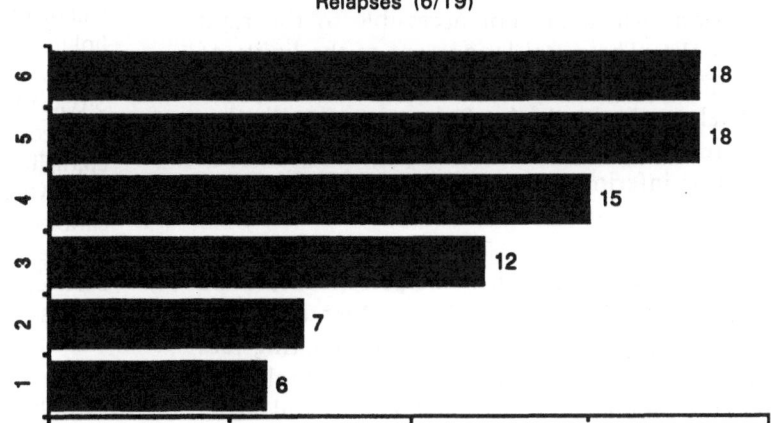

Medium-term results
Relapses (6/19)

Fig. 4. Delay between initial cryotherapy and appearance of recurrence (months)

gest being 3 years. Three recurrent tumours were treated within on year.

Of the 19 tumours treated with good initial results 6 recurred (Fig. 3). Four of these (left main bronchus, trifurcation of right upper bronchus, anterior branch of right middle bronchus, spur of the medial basal bronchus of the right lower lobe) were technically difficult to reach. The other two were extensive superficial infiltrating lesions of the left main bronchus and the apex of the right basal bronchus. The recurrences were noted up to 18 months following the initial treatment, and four occurred within one year (Fig. 4).

The treatment of recurrences was as follow : 5 cases of repeat cryosurgery of which four were alone and 1 in association with radiotherapy. This last patient had been irradiated without preliminary cryosurgery, thus the effect of this radiotherapy could not be estimated. Of the 5 patients who underwent cryosurgery for a second time 3 obtained good immediate results, 1 confirmed by biopsy and 2 at 3 and 14 months follow up.

Two tumours did not respond to a second cryosurgery, one due to difficulty of access (on the spur of the trifurcation of the right upper lobe bronchus) and the other on the anterior branch of the right upper lobe bronchus which was found not to have responded at follow up. This patient subsequently underwent an operation for a carcinoma stage $T_1 N_0$.

In summary : Up to the present, the following results have been obtained. Fifteen lesions have been controlled by cryosurgery alone, 2 following a recurrence. Of the other 5 cases additional treatment modalities had been necessary to effect a satisfactory treatment.

Other important findings to be noted are as follows.

Of the 6 patients who had a previous history of carcinoma of the airways when the superficial carcinoma was discovered 4 of these patients ultimately developed a head and neck cancer or a new bronchial carcinoma independant from the lesion treated with cryotherapy ; this recurrence occured in only one of the nine patients treated with cryosurgery who had no previous history of malignancy in the bronchi and this patient died. Overall, 3 patients died, 2 from the progression of an invasive carcinoma appearing after cryosurgery, but at a different site, and 1 from carcinoma of the prostate. No patient died from the progression of a lesion treated with cryosurgery.

Discussion

At present, cryotherapy alone appears capable of eradicating superficial bronchial carcinomas. However, with current data it is not possible to ensure good long-term results. The longest follow-up period is at present 3 years, and in our experience recurrences have often occurred after a delay of more than 1 year. It is therefore too early to regard this method as a definitive cure even for superficial lesions. The answer lies in the results of long-term endoscopic follow-up of these patients.

The method has its limitations : e.g. the accessibility of the lesions to the cryoprobe and the surface extension of the cancerous mucosa to be destroyed. The flexible cryoprobe allows access to lesions which are not accessible to the rigid cryoprobe. The distal lesions are at the limits of accessibility and are the most difficult to treat accurately and completely. It is uncertain whether the freezing obtained with the flexible cryoprobe, which is inferior to that of the rigid instrument, achieves similar complete tumour destruction, even in an easily accessible tumour treated under favourable conditions. The present results do not answer this question. The surface extension of the area to be destroyed is also a limiting factor. Very extensive tumours require multiple step by step application of cryotherapy and it is difficult to be sure that a small area of the lesion has not been missed. This type of tumour necessitates a sessional treatment and very careful follow-up.

Conclusion

The treatment of carcinoma in situ and microinvasive carcinomas of the bronchial tree is poorly classified because of the rarity of the clinical diagnosis, the uncertainty of their spontaneous evolution, their frequent association with other neoplastic manifestations of the lungs and the absence of a definite protocol for appropriate methods of treatment.

If the present good results obtained with cryotherapy are confirmed in the long-term, it may represent the therapy of choice in accessible superficial carcinomas, possibly in association with HDR brachytherapy.

References

1. Black H, Ackerman LV (1952) The importance of epidermoid carcinoma in situ in the histogenesis of carcinoma of the lung. Ann Surg 136 : 44-55
2. Auerbach O, Stout Ap, Hammond EC, Garfinkel L (1961) Changes in bronchial epithelium to cigarette smoking and in relation to lung cancer. N Engl J Med 265 : 253-267
3. Nagamoto N, Saito Y, Imai T, Suda H, Hashimoto K, Nakada T, Sato H (1986) Roentgenographically occult bronchogenic squamous cell carcinoma : location in the bronchi, depth of invasion and length of axial involvement of the bronchus. Tohoku J Exp Med 148 : 241-256
4. Nettesheim P, Klein-Szanto AJP, Marchok AC, Steele VE, Terzaghi N, Topping DC (1981) Studies of neoplastic development in respiratory tract epithelium. Arch Pathol Lab Med 105 : 1-10
5. Law MR, Hodson ME, Lennox SC (1982) Implications of histologically reported residual tumour on the bronchial margin after resection for bronchial carcinoma. Thorax 37 : 492-495
6. Cortese DA, Kinsey JH, Woolner LB, Payne LB, Sanderson DR, Fontana RS (1979) Clinical application of a new endoscopic technique for detection of in situ bronchial carcinoma. Mayo Clin Proc 54 : 636-642
7. Homasson JP, Bonniot JP, Angebault M, Renault P, Carnot F, Santelli G (1985) Fluorescence as a guide to bronchial biopsy. Thorax 40 : 38-40
8. Castella J, Puzo MC, De Las Heras P et al (1982) Método de localización del carcinoma broncogénico radiológica y endoscópicamente oculto. Arch Bronchoneumol 18 : 195-199
9. Israel L (1986) Les cancers intra-thoraciques. Flammarion medecine-sciences. Paris, pp. 73-74
10. Mason MK, Jordan JW (1982) Outcome of carcinoma in situ and early invasive carcinoma of the bronchus. Thorax 37 : 453-456
11. Shapshay Sm, Beamis JF (1989) Use of CO_2 laser. Chest 95 : 449-456
12. Hayata Y, Kato H, Konaka C, Ono J, Takizaiwa N (1982) Hematoporphyrin derivative and laser photoradiation in the treatment of lung cancer. Chest 81 : 269-277
13. Kato H, Konaka C, Kawate N, Shinohara H, Kinoshita K, Noguchi N, Ootomo S, Hayata Y (1986) Five-year disease-free survival of a lung cancer patient treated only by photodynamic therapy. Chest 90 : 768-770
14. Cortese DA (1986) Bronchoscopic photodynamic therapy of early lung cancer. Chest 90 : 629-631
15. Walsh TE, McCarrick JP, Sen RP (1990) Electrocautery resection of tracheobronchial neoplasms. Chest 98 : 132
16. Infeld M, Gerblich A, Subramanyan S, Whitlesey D (1988) Focus of bronchial carcinoma in situ eradicated by endobronchial biopsy. Chest 94 : 1107-1109
17. Ozenne G, Vergnon JM, Blanc-Jouvan F, Roullier A, Courty G, Taulelle M (1990) Cryothérapie des carcinomes in situ ou microinvasifs de l'arbre trachéobronchique. Cryothérapie : 7-10

Pleural and lung cryobiopsies during thoracoscopy

Jean-Paul Homasson and Nicholas J. Bell

Even if thoracoscopy is a well known technique used for the diagnosis of pleural lesions, the utilization of freezing techniques in chest medicine is more recent. Nevertheless, cryotherapy through rigid or flexible bronchoscopy is routinely used in the treatment of tracheo-bronchial strictures. The haemostatic, anti-inflammatory and analgesic properties of ice have been recognized for several centuries. The recent use of cryotherapy by means of a miniature crysprobe opens the field to wider applications of this technique where biopsy specimens are required. The renewed interest in the use of thoracoscopy as a diagnostic and therapeutic tool provides an opportunity to use cryotherapy to take biopsy specimens during the procedure [1].

Material

Thoracoscopy

There is no specific equipment needed to carry out cryobiopsies. It is simply necessary to use trocars with a diameter sufficiently large to allow the passage of the cryoprobe. We use the Wolf thoracoscope (Knittlingen - Germany) which consists of trocars with blunt conical tips of between 5 and 7 mm in diameter with lenses of 7 mm diameter and about 360 mm long allowing a vision of 180°, 130° and 90°. The biopsy forceps with cutting jaws and a double curette may be used ; the eyepiece enabling a sample to be taken under direct vision (Fig. 1).

Cryo unit

The freezing of lung and pleural tissues is achieved by means of a rigid cryoprobe Erbe (Tubingen — Germany) or with a semi rigid cryoprobe DATE (La Motte d'Aveillans — France). These probes are exactly the same as those used in bronchial cryotherapy only shorter, measuring 30 mm long with a diameter of 3 mm. The entire probe is insulated except for the distal 1 cm. These probes employ the Joule-Thomson effect (cooling of a gas on sudden expansion from a high to a low pressure region), and use nitrous oxide as a coolant source. The temperature obtained at the tip of the cyroprobe is − 80° C but tissues are frozen at − 30° C or − 40° C.

To monitor the tissue freezing we use, with the French probe (DATE) an impedancemetric method, which seems, at the present time, to be

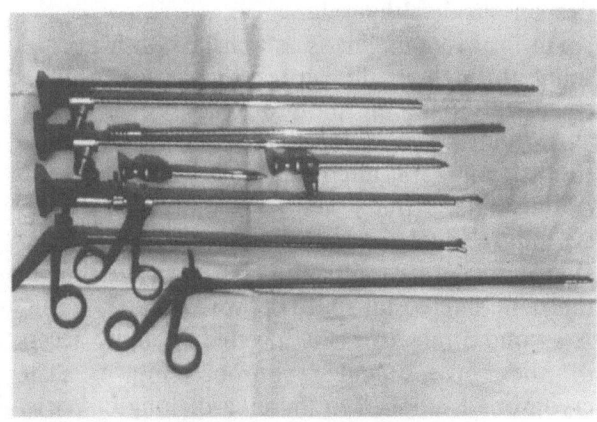

Fig. 1. Wolf thoracoscope with forceps

the most efficient (it measures the variations of resistance of tissues during the freeze-thaw cycle). It is known that extracellular crystallisation of tumour or healthy tissue (except bones) occurs at about 500 kilo ohms (KΩ). One electrode is represented by the tip of the cryoprobe and the other is either an electrode from an ECG machine or else a metal pad as used in surgery in conjunction with diathermy.

Method

Preparation of the patient

The preparation is the same as that required for a normal thoracoscopic examination. Preoperative investigations include an ECG, arterial blood gases and clotting time. We also include an HIV test when there is sufficient doubt concerning the nature of the pathology. A pneumothorax is created at the outset of the procedure by introducing one or two litres of air into the pleural cavity. If there is a pleural effusion present this is drained first. After this a check chest X-ray is taken or else a CT scan is carried out. Parietal lesions are often more clearly seen when the lung is collapsed. At this point one can also assess the best point of entry for the trocar, sometimes anteriorly but more often in the mid-axillary line.

The procedure is carried out in the usual way after premedication with Flunitrazepam, adding Pethidine if talcum powder is to be inserted into the pleural space. The intercostal space is anaesthetized with 2% Lignocaine. The patient lies on the healthy side.

An intravenous line is established with normal saline throughout the entire procedure as well as electrocardiographic monitoring.

A 7 mm trocar is introduced, generally between the 4th and 5th intercostal spaces in the mid-axillary line. After visual inspection of the cavity, any residual fluid is aspirated, a second incision is made several centimeters away, either in the same intercostal space or in the one adjacent. A second 5 mm trocar is inserted to allow access of the forceps and cyroprobe (Fig. 2). The cryoprobe is applied to the area of lung or parietal pleura to be biopsied by direct vision with the thoracoscope through the large trocar. The area is frozen, and this freezing causes a light mist. The freezing phase lasts about 45 s. Tissues in

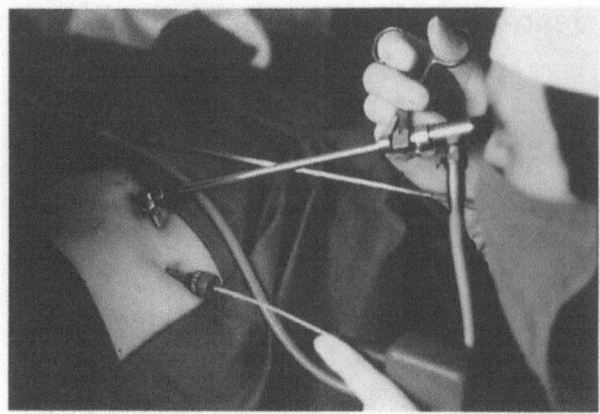

Fig. 2. Cryoprobe in place

contact with the ice are frozen and this is confirmed by an increase in electrical resistance measured at the tip of the cryoprobe of approximately 300-400 KΩ. The size of the frozen area is about 0.5 sq cm × 3 mm in depth. Thawing is almost immediate and the probe is released from the tissue. As soon as the cryoprobe is removed, the biopsy is taken. The forceps can easily catch hold of hardened frozen lung tissue at the edge of the small crater formed by the freezing process. Specimens are taken and placed in Bouin's liquid at ambient temperature. Again the cryoprobe is inserted to freeze another area. Sometimes the biopsy produces a small haemorrhage which may be easily controlled by further freezing.

At the end of the procedure, in patients with reccurent pleurisy, talc is applied to the pleural surfaces to obtain good adhesion and a 3 to 6 mm chest tube is left in place with constant aspiration at -20 or -30 cm H_2O. A chest X-ray examination is done 2 hours after the biopsy specimens were taken and repeated daily until removal of the tube. The biopsy specimen may be taken under direct vision through only one trocar (7 mm), provided it is taken within 30 seconds of freezing the tissue.

Results

Clinical results

This technique gives good results. Failures occur only when the pleura are very thickened and the lung tissue cannot be reached. The biopsy of the parietal pleura is not painful partly due to the anaesthetic effect of freezing. This has been confirmed by taking two pleural biopsies, one from a frozen area and another without freezing. The biopsy taken without freezing produces pain especially when it is taken from apparently normal pleura. Parietal pleural polypoid lesions are usually painless when biopsied but they tend to bleed, but with a cryobiopsy the freezing exerts a haemostatic effect. A lung biopsy is always painless. We have not encountered any major haemorrhage with this technique although sometimes there is a little bleeding which may be easily controlled with several freeze cycles applied directly to the bleeding site and also to the surrounding tissues. The fact that no air escapes during the biopsy is an advantage and the reinflation of the lung has never been prolonged beyond what one would normally expect after a pneumothorax.

Histopathological findings

Cryobiopsies of pleura and lungs produce perfectly adequate samples for light microscopy. The biopsies are taken immediately after freezing and are then rapidly fixed. This produces good specimens which are well preserved and are of equal quality as those taken by classical endoscopic or surgical methods. The technique may be used to diagnose an invasive neoplasm (Fig. 3), silicosis (Fig. 4) and may also be used to establish an opportunist infection in HIV (Fig. 5).

Light microscopy reveals a normal lung structure, however in electron microscopy, even with good fixation various changes are seen at the air-blood barrier which may constitute a contra indication to this type of biopsy if electron microscopy is envisaged to study the fine detail of lung tissue.

The lesions encountered vary in severity depending on which areas are studied even on the same field of view — this variation in severity may be explained by the relative distance of the lesion from the cryoprobe when it was applied to the tissue for freezing. The changes affect both the alveolar cells as well as the interstitial cells. Type 2 pneumocytes which are easily recognizable due to their osmophilic bodies appear more vulnerable than the type 1 pneumocytes where the cytoplasm appears better preserved.

The cytoplasm of these type 2 pneumocytes appears condensed and thus is dense to electrons. The edge of the cytoplasm appears indistinct (Fig. 6) and some of the cells are separated from their basal membranes (Fig. 7). In the interstitial layer the interalveolar septima are thickened by oedema. One also sees changes to the endothelial cells with turgid cytoplam and swollen mitochondria (Fig. 8). All these changes indicate marked damage to the blood-air barrier.

Discussion

As we know, thoracoscopy has two main indications : diagnostic and therapeutic. Cyrobiopsies are used for diagnosis but the effects of cold also have an analgesic and haemostatic effect. The analgesic effect of freezing has already been discussed in a previous chapter [2, 3, 4]. The haemostatic effect is useful to control any small bleed that may occur during the biopsy.

Biopsies of the visceral pleura are often difficult to achieve with forceps due to the soft nature of the underlying lung tissue — diathermy forceps may be used but the level of current is sometimes difficult to assess as the tissue may be burnt and rendered useless for histological study. There is also an added risk of secondary haemorrhage from the scar. However the effect of freezing provides a hardened tissue area which is easier to grasp with forceps.

As far as air leakage is concerned we can only hypothesise as to why this does not occur after cryobiopsy. We assume that under the scar formed by freezing the tissue heals and is reconstituted as seen in a bronchus treated with freezing and this prevents air leakage. The use of larger diameter cryoprobes with large jawed forceps could overcome the technical failures encountered with thickened pleura.

When per-bronchial endoscopic biopsies have failed to establish a diagnosis this technique offers a good alternative before an explorative thoracotomy is carried out, particularly for the pneumoconioses and pulmonary infections associated with HIV.

Conclusion

This technique appears to have several advantages. The analgesic effect of ice allows one to take several biopsy specimens without pain. The risk of haemorrhage or of air escaping seems to be reduced. Finally, with light microscopy, the quality of the biopsy specimen is better than that found using electrocoagulation, but the damage caused by freezing is well seen under electron

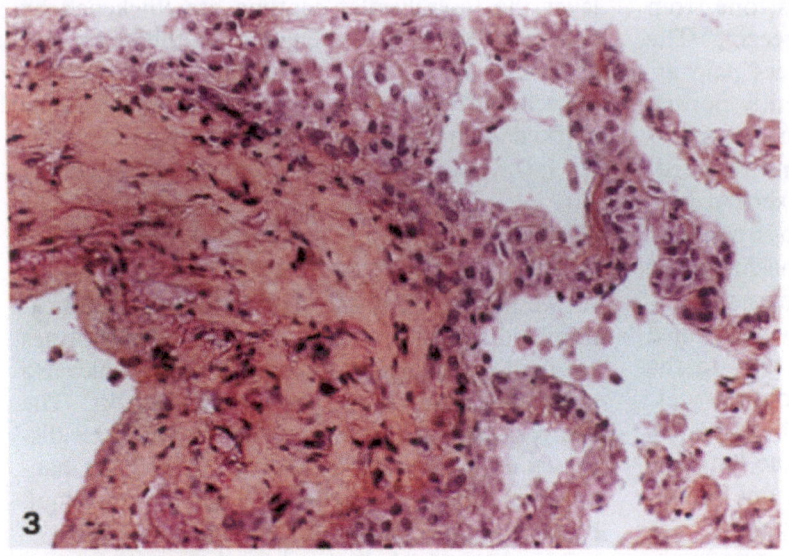

Fig. 3. Adenocarcinoma. Lung biopsy specimen showing tumour cells in the alveolar wall

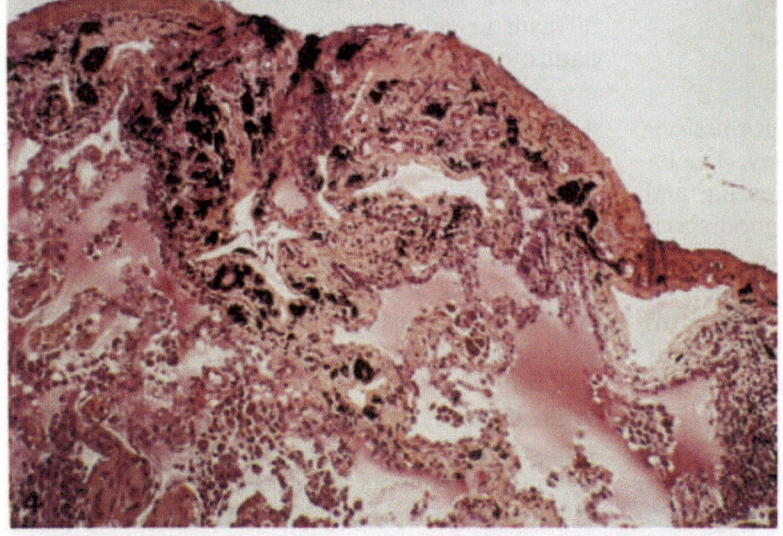

Fig. 4. Thickened pleura. Dust deposits characteristic of pneumoconiosis

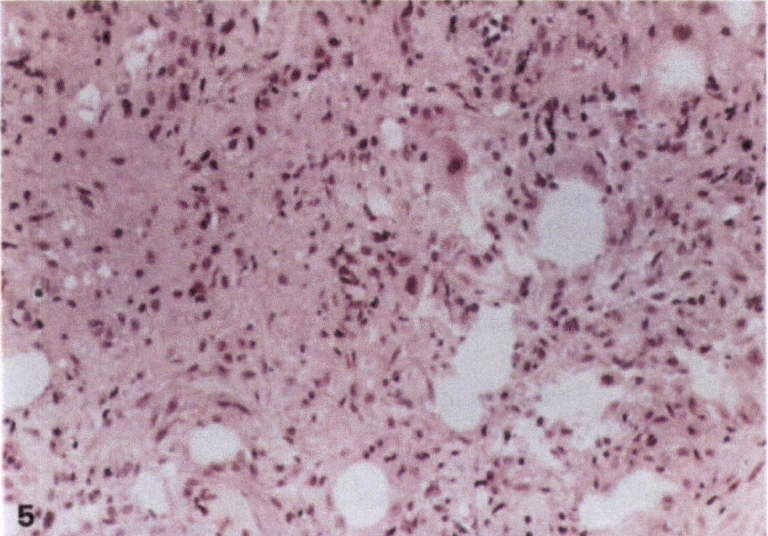

Fig. 5. Pneumonia with cytomegalovirus (CMV) showing viral inclusion bodies

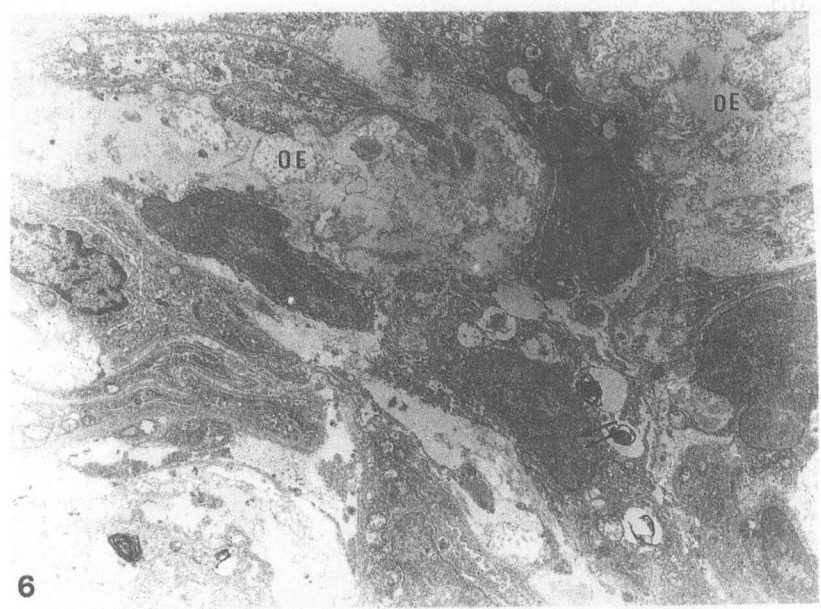

Fig. 6 Alveolar walls. Type 2 pneumocytes with degenerative changes (╱) (condensed cytoplasm — significant interstitial oedema) (OE) E.M. × 3900

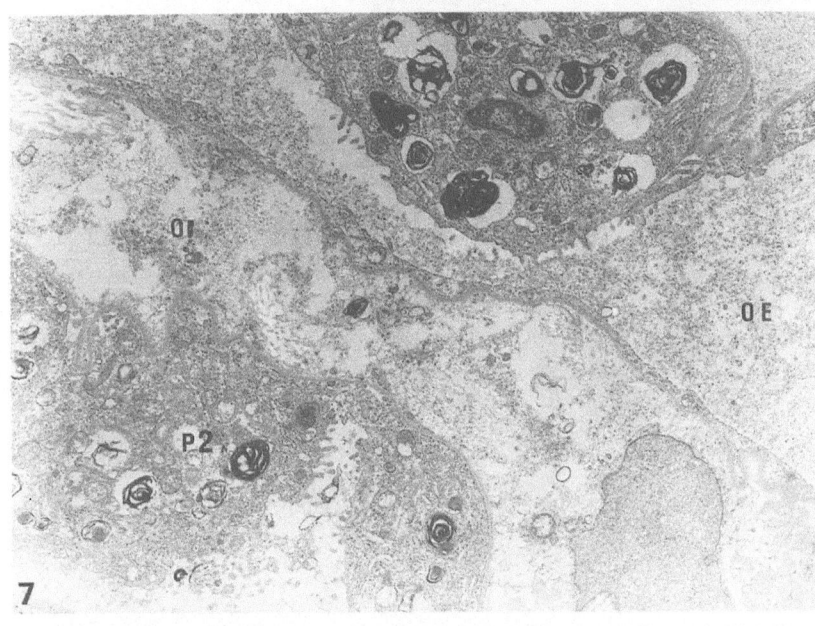

Fig. 7. Type 2 pneumocyte (P2) showing changes to the cytoplasm with interstitial oedema (OI) and alveolar oedema (OE). E.M. × 4500

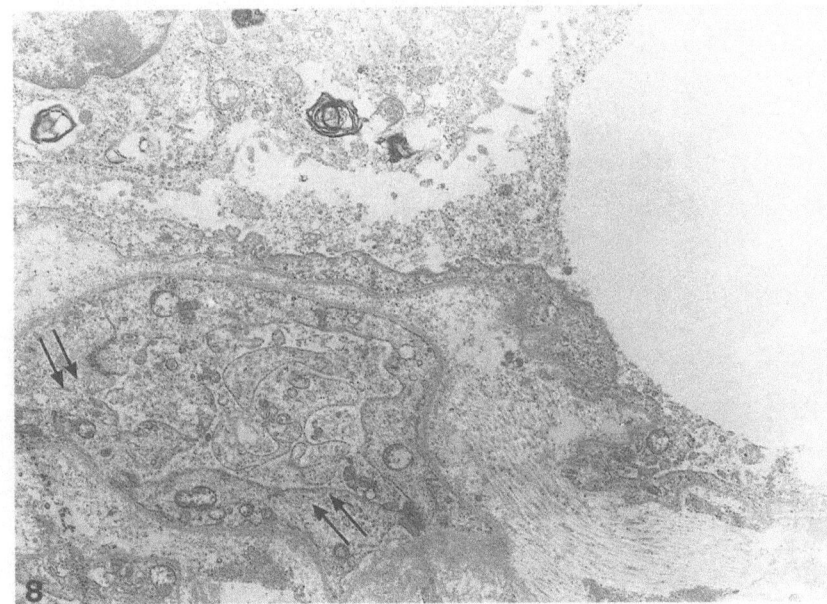

Fig. 8. Turgid endothelial cells of capillary with swollen mitochondria (╱). E.M. × 5900

microscopy after a simple freeze-thaw cycle which confirms the effect of cryotherapy, namely tissue destruction.

Acknowledgements. We thank Pierre Renault, Bernadette Rain and Françoise Lange for the histological specimens.

References

1. Bonniot JP, Homasson JP, Roden S, Angebault M, Renault P (1989) Pleural and lung cryobiopsies during thoracoscopy. Chest 95 : 492-493

2. Evans PJD (1981) Cryoanalgesia : the application of low temperatures to nerves to produce anaesthesia or analgesia. Anaesthesia 36 : 1003-1013

3. Glynn CJ, Lloyd JW, Barnard JWD. Cryoanalgesia in the management of pain after thoracotomy. Thorax 35 : 325-327

4. Maiwand O, Makey AR (1981) Cryoanalgesia for relief of pain after thoracotomy. Br Med J 282 : 1749-1750

Cryoanalgesia for control of post thoracotomy pain

M. Omar Maiwand

Management of post operative pain following thoracotomy can be a major problem due to extent and nature of the surgical procedure. Different methods of pain control have been tried [1-3] but there is no universal single regime which provides effective analgesia while being devoid of adverse effects.

In the last few years a new analgesic technique has been evolved which may lead to considerable changes in the way both acute and chronic pain is treated. This technique is known as cryoanalgesia : controlled application of local cooling to nerves [4].

The analgesic effect of freezing has been known from early times. This was recorded first by Hippocrates in about (400BC). John Hunter in 1777 observed the analgesic effects of cold during animal experiments.

The French Military Surgeon, Larrey, utilised the effects of freezing to perform painless amputations during the retreat from Moscow in 1812. Trendelenburg in 1918 demonstrated that nerve function was interrupted by freezing and was impressed by the excellent regeneration which followed.

Rapid technical progress in the use of cryoanalgesia occurred after 1961 when the American Neurosurgeon, Cooper, and his colleague, Lee, first produced a liquid nitrogen probe to control the tremor of Parkinson's disease.

In 1964 the South African Ophtalmic Surgeon, Amoils, produced a ball-point probe for ophtalmic surgical procedures using CO_2 or nitrous oxide gas and employing the Joule-Thompson principle, whereby high pressure gas is allowed to expand within the probe and causes rapid cooling to approximately — 60° C at the tip. Since then this principle has been applied to different branches of medicine to treat a variety of conditions [5]. This has been maid possible by the technical advances in the design of the probe which enables the nerve to be located and frozen in the tissue without surgical exposure.

Cryo-effect

A peripheral nerve consists of a number of bundles of fascicles of nerve fibres. A fascicle contains — myelinated and unmyelinated axons which are surrounded and supported by connective tissue sheaths (Endoneurium). Axons may give off one or more collateral branches. Each nerve fibre is enclosed by perineurium, a strong fibrous sheath which protects the axon and serves as a diffusion barrier between nerve fibres. Bundles are usually arranged in groups which are embedded in epineurium [6]. Cooling of peripheral nerve fibres produces a prolonged reversible block of conduction. It is generally agreed that this occurs at temperatures between — 5° C and — 20° C [7].

The anatomical and biochemical changes which occur during freezing are due to the removal of pure water from the cell and the formation of ice crystals [8]. This causes hypertonicity of intra and extra cellular fluid [9] membrane rupture due to rapid water loss [10] and damage to cell proteins [11]. Formation of large ice crystals causes physical destruction of cells and ischaemic necrosis [12].

Cooling to temperatures below − 20° C has no further advantage. In addition once the nerve is frozen to this temperature, no further benefit will be produced by prolonging the exposure, lowering the temperature or repeating the freezing cycles [13].

Freezing of a peripheral nerve causes disintegration of the axon cylinders and myelin sheaths and Wallerian degeneration occurs distal to the cryolesion [14].

The neural connective tissue sheaths, perineurium and epineurium are, however, not similarly affected by freezing and this facilitates regeneration of nerve fibre [15] no apparent proximal degeneration being seen. The time for recovery depends on the distance from the cryolesion to the end organs and is usually at the rate of about 1 mm per day [16]. The inflammatory response to cold and subsequent fibrosis may modify or interfere with the rate and range of recovery.

Technique of freezing and positioning of chest tube

A postero-lateral thoracotomy, which is a common approach for intra-thoracic procedures, normally gives an easy access to the intercostal nerves. At the end of the procedure, prior to closure of the chest, the intercostal nerve should be located and seen clearly. Local peeling of the parietal pleura is advisable in patients with thickened pleura where identification of the intercostal nerve is not possible.

The probe should be placed under direct vision on the nerve, proximal to the collateral branch (Fig. 1). Care must be taken that the ice ball area should cover the whole of the nerve. To achieve maximum physical effect and sufficient drop of temperature at the probe tip, the nitrous oxide cylinder must have enough pressure (600 K-Pascal).

The development of a curved cryoprobe has facilitated the positioning of the probe. This has a trochar tip and a strong stem which allows accurate anatomical access to the nerve under direct vision.

The intercostal nerve at the thoracotomy space and one intercostal nerve above and two intercostal nerves below the space should be frozen for 30 seconds only.

The probe should be allowed to defrost in situ prior to removal, otherwise the property of cryoadhesion may damage the nerve if the probe is removed without allowing time to defrost.

Tissue temperature recording made on 100 consecutive patients during the procedure showed a mean temperature of approximately − 20° C [17].

To obtain maximum benefit from the cryotherapy, the chest drains should be placed within cyro-treated spaces. To ensure this, the chest tube may have to be placed a space or two higher than the routinely used position.

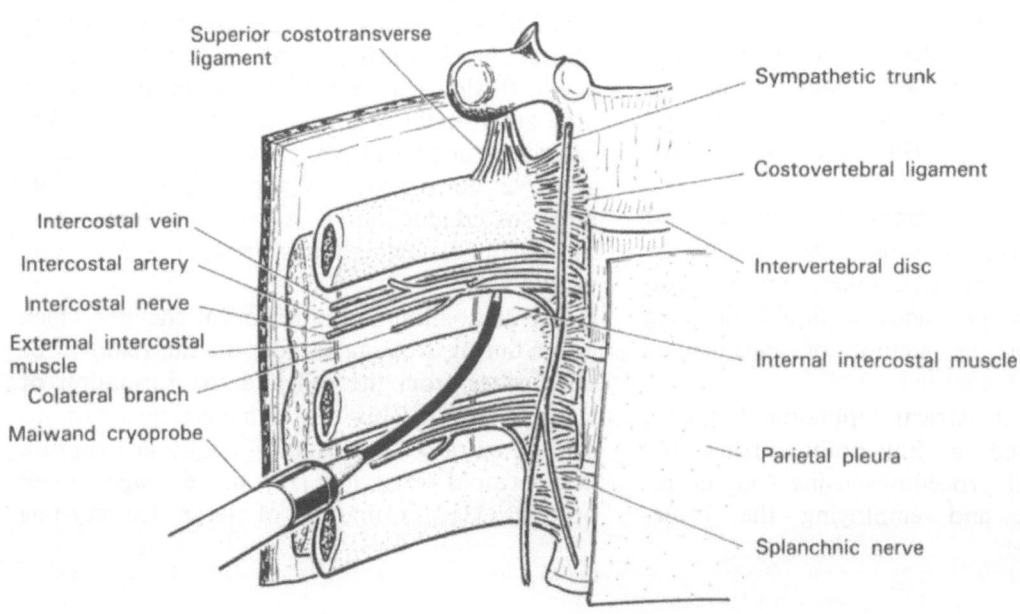

Fig. 1. Diagram showing precise positioning of the cryoprobe on the intercostal nerve proximal to the collateral branch prior to freezing

Indications for cryoanalgesia

Experience with over 1000 patients who had cryoanalgesia for control of post-thoracotomy pain since 1982, suggests that cryoanalgesia is an ideal method of pain control especially for :

1. Elderly patients, whose early mobility is of utmost importance for quick recovery from major thoracic surgery.

2. Patients with poor respiratory function tests, where full co-operation and participation to physiotherapy is required to assist in the re-expansion of the remaining lung and to prevent further complications.

3. Patients where early removal of the chest drains is essential to recover from their surgical procedure.

4. Where a tumour is infiltrating the chest wall and mediastinal structures.

5. Left thoraco-laparotomy incisions.

Effectiveness of physiotherapy after cryoanalgesia

Effective physiotherapy and early mobilisation is very important in the prevention of post operative complications, such as partial or total lung collapse, pneumonia, poor venous return, deep vein thrombosis and an ultimate sequela, pulmonary emboli.

To achieve this, physiotherapists need the co-operation of the patient. This is not possible if the patients have not received effective analgesia to control the pain which normally accompanies the long incision and prolonged retraction of the thoracotomy wound. Placing the chest tube within a small intercostal space also causes severe pain. Various pain control methods have been used, most commonly narcotic analgesics which are given prior to physiotherapy, but may have the disadvantage of respiratory depression, drowsiness and nausea.

We studied three groups of 100 consecutive patients to evaluate the effectiveness of postoperative pain relief from Cryoanalgesia, Injection of local anaesthetic or Narcotic analgesia [18].

Group 1 — were treated with cryoanalgesia.

Group 2 — were given local anaesthetic. Injection of Bupivacaine directly to the intercostal nerve (4 ml of 0.5 % Marcain).

Group 3 — were treated conventionally with intramuscular narcotic analgesics given as required.

Cryo procedure and injection of local anaesthetic were performed by the same operator. A single physiotherapist performed physiotherapy. The Ward Staff were not informed as to which Group the patient belonged. The postoperative regimen and analgesia ordered were identical for all groups. Standard chest physiotherapy was given to all three groups ; the duration and type of treatment were identical across all groups. Results of the study are shown in Tables 2 and 3.

Table 1. Composition of three groups of 100 patients undergoing major thoracic surgery receiving different types of analgesia post-operatively

		Group I : Cryo-analgesia	Group II : Marcain Injection	Group III : Conventional Narcotic Analgesia
Sex	Male	84	70	67
	Female	16	30	33
Mean age (years)		55	54	55
Age range		6-86	19-79	20-77
Operation				
Lung resection		68	61	60
Oesophageal disease		11	24	24
Pleurectomy		11	8	4
Pulmonary decortication		4	4	8
Mediastinal pathology		6	3	2

Table 2. Findings in the three groups

	Group I	Group II	Group III
Patients with severe pain (%)	9	84	89
Patients with mild pain (%)	12	16	11
Patients free of pain (%)	79	0	0
Mean No. of narcotic injections required	1.53	5.1	5.5
Patients needing oral analgesia (%)	18	75	73
Duration of oral analgesia (weeks)	4 to 8	24+	24+
Patients needing post-operative bronchoscopy (%)	0	4	4
Patients needing nasopharyngeal suction (%)	4	15	17
Early post-operative segmental or subsegmental collapse of lung confirmed by chest x-ray (%)	8	20	18
Drop in systolic blood pressure in the early post-operative period (> 80 mm Hg) (%)	0	3	0

Table 3. Pain relief obtained following cryoanalgesia

No. of patients	600
Percentage of patients free from post-operative discomfort	83
Percentage of patients with mild post-operative pain	10
Percentage of patients with severe postoperative pain	7
Mean duration of analgesia (days)	27
Mean duration of numbness (days)	38

Table 4. Analgesic requirement post-operatively

No. of patients	600
Mean no. of narcotic injections per patient (0-48 hour) post-operatively	0.87
Percentage of patients needing oral analgesia post-operatively	21
Mean duration of requirement for oral analgesia* (week)	3-6

* The analgesics given were daraphen (Distalgesic UK) and acetaminophen (Panadol)

Results and comment

Cryoanalgesia provided very effective post-thoracotomy control of pain in about 80 % of patients. Table 4 and Figure 2 show detailed results of the effectiveness of cryoanalgesia in a further 600 patients.

The chief advantage of cryoanalgesia is usually the pain free area around the thoracotomy wound. The placing of the chest tube in the cryo-treated spaces, allows handling and dressing of the wound around the tube site without undue pain and discomfort to the patient. In addition, because of the avoidance of the drowsiness and respiratory depression induced by narcotics, the patients are alert and co-operative, keen and willing to follow the instructions of the physiotherapist and the nurses — which in turn assists in reducing post-operative complications. For example, we showed that early post-operative segmen-

tal or subsegmental collapse of the lung was seen in only 8 % of the cryo group, compared to a 20 % incidence with the alternative methods [18]. The obvious advantages of early mobilisation and reduced chest complications with cryoanalgesia enabled us to accept a large percentage of older patients for surgical treatment (Fig. 2) who generally responded in the same manner as the younger age groups [17].

However, there are some disadvantages to the technique. A small percentage of patients complain of prolonged anaesthesia, or paraesthesia. In the few who complained of pain its site was usually related to a single nerve, which presumably had been inadequately frozen. The time of onset of the pain was too early to suggest neuroma formation. Early post-operative back pain of varying severity was mentioned by a significant number of patients. The pain in this instance is due to the straining of the ligaments of the costo-vertebral and costo-transverse joints by

Percentage

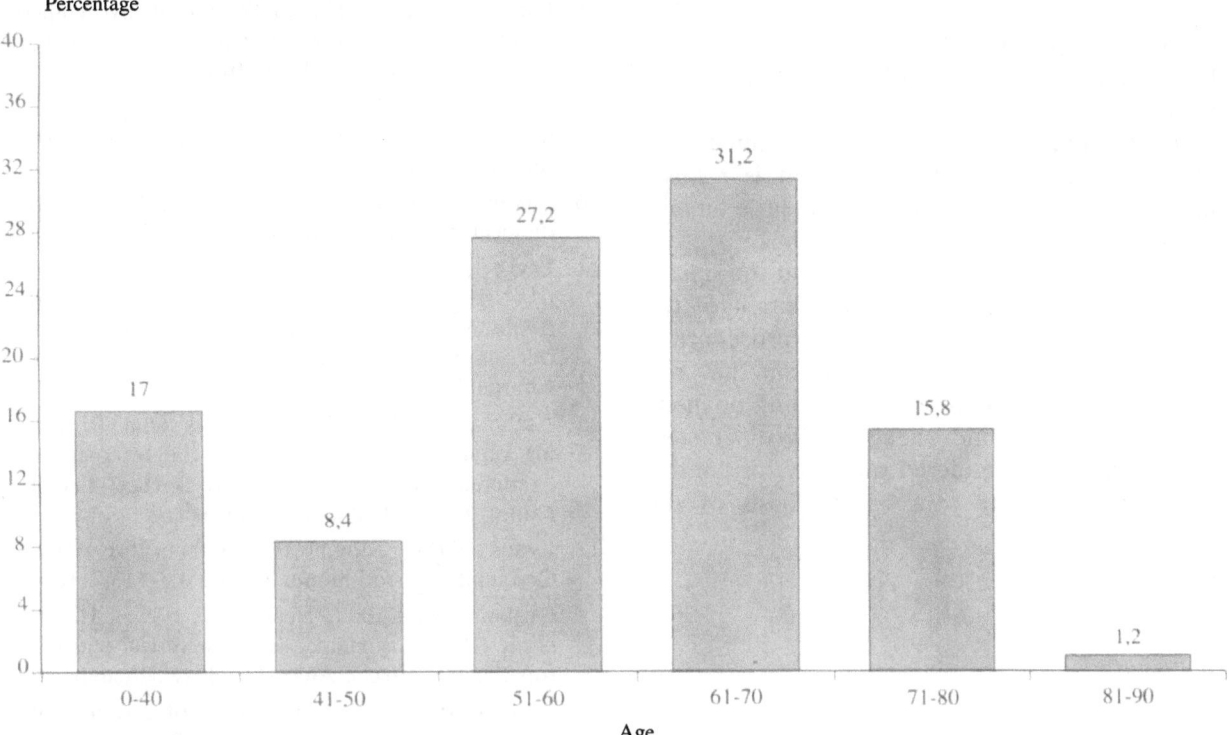

Fig. 2. Age distribution

retraction of the intercostal spaces and lateral positioning of the patient on the table. This area is supplied by the posterior primary rami of the intercostal nerves which are not blocked by the cryoprobe.

An unpleasant rigid feeling of the chest wall was reported in about 20 % of patients and bulging of the ipsilateral abdominal wall occured in a significant number of patients implying total block of the intercostal nerves. These findings disappear with the regeneration of the nerves.

A disturbing complaint was the loss of sensation in the nipple area and loss of response to mammary stimuli in four female patients. Even though the sensation returned subsequently and recovery was complete, we generally avoid freezing the 4th and 5th intercostal nerves. Since the early study we recommend that this suggestion be followed when treating young female patients.

It is also our observation that even though two 30 second cycles of freezing application to each intercostal nerve provided effective pain relief, the regeneration of the nerve took longer than expected (6-9 months). Hence we have modified our original technique to a single freeze cycle of 30 seconds only to each intercostal nerve, which provides similar analgesia but shortens the regeneration period.

Of other methods used to alleviate pain, Bupivacaine administered by thoracic extra epidural catheter [19] gives good pain relief but causes hypotension, necessitating additional colloid infusion and may lead to muscle weakness and urinary retention. Opiate drugs administered by the epidural route are free of the side effects described above, and a single injection of between 2 mg and 4 mg of morphine may produce profound analgesia for up to 12 hours. However, late onset of respiratory depression may sometimes be seen with epidural opiates and should therefore be restricted to patients who can be monitored in a high dependency or Intensive Care Unit. A skilled operator and trained nursing staff are required for the provision/management of epidural analgesia, and this along with the restrictions and the adverse effects aforementioned limits its use [20].

Intravenous injection of narcotic drugs by a mechanical pump or by a patient controlled analgesia apparatus has been shown to be a very effective method [21] but in the context of thoracic surgery patients the adverse effects, such as drowsiness and respiratory depression suggest caution in this method being used routinely.

Non narcotic analgesics, even though free from the above side effects, may not provide adequate/effective analgesia in this group of patients.

In summary, the current review has reinforced our original opinion that in the treatment of post-thoracotomy pain, cryoanalgesia offers advantages not achieved by other methods.

This technique only adds about 10 min to the total operating time. The equipment is robust, relatively inexpensive and needs little maintenance.

There have been no ill — effects to the operator, assistant or nursing staff as a result of the use of cyrosurgical equipment. The procedure is simple to perform, non-traumatic and has not been shown to cause increased bleeding or interference with wound healing. We suggest cryoanalgesia be considered routinely for control of post-thoracotomy pain on the basis of the above discussion.

References

1. Moore DC (1975) Intercostal nerve block for postoperative somatic pain following surgery of the thorax and upper abdomen. Br J Anaesth 47 : 284-288
2. Griffiths DPG, Diamond AW, Cameron JD. Postoperative extradural analgesia following thoracic surgery. A feasibility study. Br J Anaesth 47 : 48-55
3. James EC, Colberg HL, Iwen GW, Gellatly TA, Forks G (1981) Epidural analgesia for postthoracotomy patients. J Thorac Cardiovasc Surg 82 : 898-903
4. Lloyd JW, Barnard JDW, Glynn CJ (1976) Cryoanalgesia — a new approach to pain relief. Lancet 11 : 932-934
5. Ablin RJ (1980) Handbook of cryosurgery. Marcel Dekker Inc., New York, 109-311
6. Burge P (1990) Peripheral nerve injuries. Surgery 86 : 2059-2063
7. Gaster Rn, Davidson TM, Rand RW, Fonkalstrud EW (1971) Comparison of nerve regeneration rates following controlled freezing or crushing. Arch Surg 103 : 378-383
8. Evans PJD (1981) The application of low temperatures to nerves to produce anaesthesia or analgesia. Anaesthesia 36 : 1003-1013
9. Farrant J (1965) Mechanism of cell damage during freezing and thawing and its prevention. Nature 205 : 1284-1287
10. Litvan GG (1972) Mechanism of cryoinjury in biological systems. Cryobiology 9 : 182-191
11. Levitt J, Dear J (1970) The role of membrane proteins in freezing injury and resistance. In : Wolstenholme GEW, O'Connor M (eds) The frozen cell : a Ciba Foundation symposium. London : Churchill, 148-174
12. Asahina E. Cellular injury and resistance to freezing organisms : Proceedings of the International Conference on Low Temperature Science, 2, Hokkaido, Japan, Hokkaido University
13. Evans PJD, Lloyd JW, Green CJ (1980) Cryoanalgesia technique. Lancet 1 : 1188-1189
14. Heckman H, Katz J, Nelwon W, Powell H, Myers R (1980) Cryoanalgesia : biophysical and neuropathologic effects. Anaesthesiology 52 (suppl) 233
15. Barnard JDW (1980) The effects of extreme cold on sensory nerves. Ann R Coll Surg Engl 62 : 180-187
16. Whittaker DK (1974) Degeneration and regeneration of nerves following cryosurgery. Br J Experimen Path 55 : 595-600
17. Maiwand MO, Makey AR, Rees A (1986) Cryoanalgesia after thoracotomy. J Thor Cardiovasc Surg 92 : 291-295
18. Maiwand MO, Makey AR, Sanmuganathan S (1982) Increased effectiveness of physiotherapy after cryoanalgesia following thoracotomy. Physiotherapy 68 : 288-290
19. James EC, Kolberg HL, Iwen GW, Gellatly TA, Forks G (1981) Epidural analgesia for postthoracotomy patients. J Thorac Cardiovasc Surg 82 : 898-903
20. Yeager MP, Glass DD, Neff RK, Brinck-Johnsen T (1987) Epidural anaesthesia and analgesia in high risk surgical patients. Anesthesiology 66 : 729-736
21. Fry ENS (1979) Post operative analgesia using continuous infusion of Papaveratum. Ann Royal College Surg Engl 61 : 371-373

Pulmonary cryosurgery

Liu Ping, Xu Zhong-Fa and Sun Xu-Shan

Pulmonary cryosurgery has been developed over the past twenty years by Liu Ping in China. He has designed a special L-C type lung frozen-fixation instrument which he first tested on animals in 1978. Since then it has been tested on 80 patients with various lung lesions with satisfactory results. The range of tumours treated include peripheral lung lesions measuring up to 6 cm in diameter ; unilateral or bilateral, singular or even multiple metastatic lesions of the lung, and certain benign tumours such as tuberculomas or pulmonary cystic parasitic lesions.

Cryosurgical procedure

Routine open chest surgery is performed and the mass is fully exposed. A suitably sized L-C type frozen fixation instrument is selected and placed over the mass and the surrounding tissue is protected by cotton pads. Liquid nitrogen is then poured into the cup of the instrument producing rapid freezing of the lesion to approximately — 196° C. Several freeze thaw cycles are carried out and the frozen lesion is then removed and routine closure effected. Bilateral cryosurgery has been carried out at a single operation in some instances.

Results

Table 1 shows the range of lesions treated with this method.

Table 1.

Benign disease

Condition	No. of patients
Hamartoma	2
Pseudo tumours	7
Tuberculoma	9
Pulmonary cysts	2
Lobar pneumonia	3

Malignant disease (primary)

Condition	No. of patients
Adenocarcinoma	24
Squamous cell	9
Undifferentiated	3
Unclassified	1

Malignant disease (secondary metastases)

Primary tumour type	No. of patients
Sarcomas	5
Rectal carcinoma	3
Choriocarcinoma	2
Breast cancer	3
Ovarian cancer	2
Colon cancer	1
Melanoma	1
Cervical cancer	1
Testicular cancer	1
Renal cancer	1

Immediately following treatment there were no serious complications and no fatalities. Quite marked pulmonary effusion may occur postoperatively and radiology shows a large dense shadow surrounding the resected tumour. This is thought to be a reaction to the cryosurgery and usually clears 10-14 days later. Three cases of pneumothorax occured 9-27 days following cryosurgery which resolved with drainage.

Conclusion

This form of treatment is of interest as it has been developed as an alternative to local surgical resection of lung masses. The author claims that it is superior to surgical resection in selected cases and he claims improved survival in cases of primary and secondary lung cancer compared to conventional Western therapy.

It has to be said that less invasive and less aggressive treatment may be advocated by doctors in the West for some of the conditions listed in Table 1 which have been treated by this remarkable technique of pulmonary cryosurgery.

Nevertheless it merits inclusion in a book of this nature if only to complete the catalogue of mankind's endeavours to treat lung pathology with cold.

Index

Achevé d'imprimer par Corlet, Imprimeur, S.A.
14110 Condé-sur-Noireau (France)
N° d'Éditeur : 635 - N° d'Imprimeur : 5870 - Dépôt légal : décembre 1992
Imprimé en C.E.E.